# You Are the Spark

## Motivational Essays to Support Your Fitness Journey

Beth Oldfield

Prominence Publishing

www.prominencepublishing.com

The author can be reached as follows:

Website: betholdfield.ca

Facebook: Beth Oldfield_Fitness

Instagram: @betholdfield_fitness

You Are the Spark/Oldfield, Beth. -- 1st ed.

ISBN: 978-1-988925-82-0

# AUTHOR'S NOTE

One of my greatest strengths as a fitness instructor is my ability to tailor my large group exercise classes to individual participants. While personal training remains near and dear to my heart, I have been able to inspire and positively affect the lives of far more people through my line dance, tabata, Essentrics®, yoga, muscle conditioning and aerobics classes than I could have ever done through one-on-one training. Group fitness is magical in the way that it lifts our collective spirits and motivates us to move. My entire raison d'être as a Fitness Professional is to help my students to be the best that they can be in body, mind, and soul. Each day I am aiming to deliver an even better class than I did the day before so that my students can reach their potential.

I started my blog in April of 2015 to provide feedback based on what I was seeing within the various groups that I lead. The truth is there was never enough time to answer questions and concerns in great depth before or after class. I was careful to never mention names within my posts, but I took my cues from you, my students, when deciding what topics needed to be addressed so that you could improve your performance and your health.

I recently launched my new website at betholdfield.ca and instead of simply transferring over 400 blog posts to the new location, I decided to turn them into a book to inspire and lead you through your fitness journey. You will see posts from 2015 through to 2020 on topics that are loosely divided into sections to help you to find the exact motivation needed on any given day.

Diane Ferland, (one of my longest attending members) once told me that I should turn my blog into a motivational coffee table book. I honestly never thought I would have enough material. I guess I have had lots to say. Thanks for planting the seed, Diane.

Here is my first blog post on April 18th, 2015.

# Getting Started

April 18, 2015

If you want to know the truth, I am tired of talking to myself. That is why I am jumping into this world of blogging. I have so much information to share, on so many subjects, that this blog will be about a diverse range of subjects.

I have over fifteen years of teaching experience in the fitness industry. I teach yoga, muscle conditioning, stability ball, step, stretching and line dance. I am also a personal trainer. My focus is on creating balance in the body and mind. The success of my students gives me such joy. I absolutely love what I do each day!

You should know that I am also an avid reader and writer looking to complete and publish my first book. I write both fiction and non-fiction.

I have an allergy to gluten which manifests as dermatitis herpetiformis (DH). This has forced me to learn a whole new way of cooking and living.

Together with my amazing husband of 26 years, we have designed and built two houses (with our own hands) and enjoy remote, country living at its best.

I am a proud mother of three adult children who have taught me many lessons over the years. I initially intended to teach

English and MRE (Moral and Religious Education) to secondary students but once I became a mother, I decided to stay home and raise my beautiful kids. Still feeling the need to teach, I studied at night toward becoming a fitness instructor with the YMCA. I achieved this goal in 1998 and have loved leading adults towards improved health ever since.

My hope is that by sharing my personal experiences, I can help people to be the best that they can be, in all aspects of life.

Wish me luck!

# FOREWORD

I cannot think of anyone who embodies the qualities and values of "professionalism" more than Beth Oldfield. I have known and worked with Beth since 2009 as both a private client and as part of her group exercise classes.

I started out with Beth when I was leading a very sedentary lifestyle and weighing about 160lbs. I hired her to be my personal trainer and every month she would develop a new program based on my progress and needs. Beth did this every month for about 3 years. Did I want to give up - Yes. Did I find it challenging - always! Beth was both my inspiration and my rock. She didn't just give me exercises but helped me deal with the mental challenges of trying every day to do my program. Beth was available if I had any questions about an exercise to ensure I did it properly and was always on my team providing motivation. Beth is always smiling and laughing. She brings so much energy and enthusiasm to the class that even I find it fun. Beth spends a lot of time choosing music to go with her classes. This is incredibly important as I find it influences both my mood and how much energy I put in. Beth is constantly sharing her knowledge about how our bodies work and is vigilant to ensure that we do the exercises correctly.

Beth has always been an innovator, teacher, and motivator. She self-published an exercise book and made fitness videos to go with it, for healthy seniors with her and her husband demonstrating each exercise. She wanted to reach those people who for whatever reason could not attend a class but would benefit from an easy-to-follow exercise regime that allowed people to progress as they became more fit.

Beth has bloomed in this COVID environment - she literally turned lemons into lemonade. In a matter of a days, she had her virtual gym up and running and personally talked her many technically challenged seniors how to get on ZOOM and what to do when we get kicked off. Beth has out done herself in making her virtual classes and exercises accessible. She is constantly posting videos showing a specific exercise that she wants to ensure that we understand and are doing correctly. Like all good fitness instructors, Beth offers many ways of doing an exercise depending on your level of fitness but in a way that no one feels "less than".

However, the thing that makes Beth stand out is no matter where she is teaching - her private classes, is the close personal relationships she develops with her students. Beth knows everyone's names (over 120 students currently) and knows most of their aches and pains. It is clear to everyone that she cares deeply about the wellbeing of her students and wants us to be healthy and vibrant well into 'our older years.' Beth really understands that keeping her clients physically well is only part of wellness. Many of her clients are single due to widowhood or separation or families having left the area. She created a community in every sense of the word. People have felt connected, supported and this is all due to Beth.

Several years ago I had to have major back surgery and was unable to do much of anything for almost 2 years. Just as I was beginning to get back on my feet I fell and broke my wrist which put me out of commission for another year. Thanks to Beth, I can now reach my toes (which I didn't think I would ever do again) and I currently weight 135lbs and I play pickleball almost every day when the weather is good. Oh yes - I attend at least one of Beth's class (sometimes two) 5x's/week. She has finally won me over and I look forward to my time with her; moving my body and being with my community.

Susan Sowerby

# WHAT PEOPLE ARE SAYING...

I was fortunate enough to reconnect with Beth in August 2020, five months into the pandemic. I have taken many in person classes with Beth since 2016 so was super excited to hear she was now offering classes through her Virtual Fitness Studio! Beth arranged for me to try a couple of classes - I wasn't sure how fitness over Zoom would work. Well, it works perfectly! I immediately signed up and have exercised almost every weekday since then. Keeping active, physically and mentally, is something I need to do daily. Chair Yoga, Essentrics®, Chair Muscle and Aerobics make me feel healthy and ready to meet the day no matter how it unravels! Variety is the spice of life and Beth's classes offer so much - without these options I would likely have become very sedentary - not a good thing no matter what your age. I am motivated by Beth to keep showing up to exercise and will continue to do what is right for both my body and my mind! –Wendy Simla

There is no doubt that Beth's fitness classes have improved my health over the years. I have followed her chair muscle stretch classes for approximately 14 years now and I find that I have more energy and physical mobility than when I first started. My osteopath has been following me once every three to four months during those years because of previous hip pain and he often praises me for my improvement in posture and mobility. At my present age of 72, I feel more mentally and physically balanced than I did in my fifties. I highly recommend Beth's courses! Linda Haynes

Just a little note to thank-you and to let you know how appreciative I am for the structure and copious amount of energy, that I now have. Instead of waking up and moping around watching tv, and wallowing in self pity, because of our present limitations, I now have a reason to get up and start my day. My arms have become stronger and more toned and hopefully by summer, I will not be too self conscious of wearing sleeveless dresses. You definitely helped improve my outlook on life, and I am looking forward to a great summer. -Lisa Kalushny

I have been a member of Beth's Fitness class since I retired ten years ago. Beth is passionate about teaching fitness and her enthusiasm coupled her zany sense of humor makes the hard work of daily exercise feel like fun. Her belief that each of us has the potential to continually improve our level of fitness motivates us to reach for our personal fitness goals. Beth's knowledge of the latest techniques in fitness, provide us with the tools that we, as seniors, need to achieve our maximum level of physical fitness and overall health. -Nancy Pasquini

I am very satisfied with your classes and especially with the variety. My last bone density Xray showed that my osteopenia had not progressed for five years, though I lost 1 inch in height! Thank you for continuing to be an excellent fitness teacher during this pandemic. It has been awesome to be able to stay in shape in my own home with the personal touch, comments that assures me that you are committed and love what you are doing. -Dianne C

Beth's classes have not only improved my physical health but kept me sane during lockdown! Even though I don't know many people in the class it is good to see friendly faces and hear the conversations before each class. Beth's upbeat comments and words of encouragement have spurred me on to keep moving and keep fit as I age. I am 20 years older than Beth, so she is just a kid to me! -Janet Ankcorn

Beth's classes are wonderful in many ways. I feel fitter, looser and have better posture. Not only that but it is heartwarming to see Beth each day, always in a good mood and to see so many friends I used to see in person at the gym. Especially now with the pandemic it has been a real lifeline for me. A reason to get up in the morning! Keep up the good work. -Tish Jones

I have been with Beth for just about two years and have enjoyed every workout session with her. Beth has always showed a personal interest in each and every one of us. I used to have hip issues, but because of her Essentrics® classes I no longer have those issues. I look forward to getting up in the morning and starting my day with my workouts. -Carol Penpeck

I am not a fan of exercising, but Beth makes her fitness classes enjoyable. I am constantly impressed and motivated by how upbeat, friendly and positive she is during her sessions. -Naile Kudeki

Taking your classes this past year and a half has not only been a sanity saviour but also a body toner and muscle builder. My physio was really surprised at how strong my quads are. I feel it has helped me maintain good flexibility and endurance, not to mention to establish a morning routine that is critical in these times of Covid. Thank you from the bottom of my heart for your enthusiasm and for making these classes feel like I am part of a special group of people. -Pat Jones

I am so fortunate to be able to participate online with Beth almost daily - I have had gym memberships and taken fitness classes off and on my entire adult life and have always felt like the unfit and uncoordinated stepsister in any in person group setting. And the commitment to put a coat on and warm up the car in a snowstorm! Beth makes me feel competent, and strong, and able to do anything, and talks us through every pose, every move, and encourages me to try again another day. I have grown to love walking the dog because nothing hurts anymore. I am sleeping better at night. And I feel great. -Cindy McCuig

Beth's classes gave me back my freedom of movement! After a fall of sorts, I injured both knees and Beth introduced me to Essentrics® which healed my knees and put me onto a journey of well being! I now can garden, hike and snowshoe without pain or any discomfort! Beth virtual classes allow me to participate even if we are at the cottage! It is a great way to start the day! -Jane Cosh

I truly believe I wouldn't have come through this awful pandemic as well as I have without having Beth's classes to nourish my body and my mind. With so much sadness around her daily workouts helped me to stay focused on remaining healthy and strong for myself and my family. -Barb Redivo

Beth's methodology and personality combine to enhance my physical, intellectual and psychological well being. She uses analogies that are simple but effective. Her exercises are geared towards developing heath and agility among the young, but it is her work with the elderly where she especially shines. There, she focuses on exercises aimed at protecting her students from aches and injuries by building strength, agility, and balance. The instructions are paced to challenge our brains so as to remain sharp and focused. Her enthusiasm is infectious. Her cheerful and caring mannerism along with her thoughtful, clear and effective instructions all contribute to making each session a special part of my day. -John Pasquini

I have found Beth's virtual fitness classes very motivating. I like the fact that they are in real time, so there's no putting it off until later. They get me up and going and give a structure to my day. That is especially important during this difficult time of Covid. I am actually taking more classes now then when they were in person. Functional fitness is very important and her classes provide the training I need to stay active and independent. -Lynn Stewart

I like the French word to describe Beth. Animateur! As I get closer to my eightieth birthday, I realize that because I have chosen to stay active with Beth as my friend and mentor, I am thriving not just surviving. -Sherri Utter

Eight months into the pandemic I realized I was in trouble, both physically and mentally. Having done nothing in the way of exercise, or anything else, I knew I had to do something. But what?? Fortunately, at about this time I was introduced to Beth's virtual classes through a local church. My life has turned around thanks to Beth and her workouts. I do four a week and wouldn't dream of missing one. I am feeling so much better now in all ways. Beth is a great instructor and has something for everyone. One of her main focuses is to keep, us "oldies" in better shape. Beth is committed and dedicated. - Leslie Sparks

At 74 years old, Beth's classes have given me significantly more flexibility and   reduction in joint pain. I suffer from arthritis, and her classes get me to move all of my joints everyday, and this keeps the arthritis manageable.   Another benefit I have received has been giving me a broader range of motion, which allows me to continue to do the daily activities I enjoy doing. I feel rejuvenated after every class. Committing to doing your classes has helped me to stay active, and this is exactly what I need to remain viable. -Ralph Cosh

The best thing I ever did was to join Beth's virtual classes last year after a recommendation from a friend. I was emotionally, physically and mentally drained as a result of seven years of giving constant care to my husband who battled cancer. He passed away and the Covid lockdown was enforced. Loneliness and isolation from family and friends were overbearing and I spiralled into a deep depression. Beth's classes filled my time and gave me contact with a friendly, bubbly fitness coach. Thanks to these classes I overcame my desperate situation. I regained my physical and mental health. I look forward to each class and I love them all -Ramona

I started exercising reluctantly 20 years ago as I felt my body needed it. It was Beth's enthusiasm and encouragement that has kept me going. Then the virus shut the gym. I was not motivated to exercise at home but decided to give Beth's virtual classes a try. I am grateful that Beth has kept me going, her classes are varied, work all the muscles in our bodies and have become an essential part of my daily routine. In spite of my aging body, she is helping me to stay fit and hopefully to age backwards. -Sandy Gordon-Loiello

Beth is truly one of the most knowledgeable, helpful fitness instructors I have ever met. Not only do I appreciate her ability to do all the exercises with us while explaining in depth why its a necessary move and where it is helping to keep our body healthy, but she truly cares about not overdoing an injured part of our bodies and is sympathetic with individual needs/abilities so always gives us alternatives. As a client with rheumatoid arthritis since the age of 28, I have been committed to exercising regularly and had many opportunities to join various classes. No one has cared more about her students than Beth and her efforts to provide new movements monthly as well as her upbeat music, and lighthearted joyful conversation has kept me a loyal healthy, pain-free customer for the past eight years. Everyone should be so lucky to have Beth in their lives! -Shelley Hall

# CONTENTS

# PART ONE

# FITNESS PROGRAMS

**W**henever I meet a new client one of the first questions I am asked is, "What is the best exercise?" Over the last 20 years I have deduced that the best exercise is the one that you will do several times per week.

Mo Hagen, one of my mentors, and the Chief Operating Officer at canfitpro, (Canada's leading fitness education provider since 1993) has always maintained that the most important message we need to deliver to Canadians is that they need to sit less and move more!

According to canfitpro, to improve your cardiorespiratory fitness, you need to accumulate a minimum of 300 minutes of moderate-intensity aerobic activity per week which is about 43 minutes per day or 150 minutes of vigorous-intensity activity per week or about 22 minutes per day. To improve your strength and functional performance you need to do muscle strengthening exercises, for all the major muscle groups, on three or more days per week, and to remain flexible, you must participate in stretching activities four or more days per week.

At the time of writing and printing of this book, the world is grappling with the COVID-19 Pandemic. Most fitness facilities are closed, and a few are offering online options of their programs. I am proud to say that within days of the gym shutting its doors last March, I was able to transition all my private clients to virtual classes and in the summer of 2020, I launched Beth's Virtual Fitness Studio.

The following section offers insight into the benefits of different types of classes and training programs. I hope it helps you to find ways to move more throughout your week.

# CERTIFICATION MATTERS

April 10, 2019

If you are looking to join a gym that offers classes, don't go for the cheapest fitness facility. Instead look for a business that guarantees that their staff is highly qualified and certified. Each professional certification demands that the instructor keep learning to re-certify each year. You are putting your health in the hands of strangers and you want to know that they are going to deliver safe programming.

I'm in the business of certifying quality instructors with canfitpro. I believe that gyms should only hire qualified fitness professionals who have kept their certification up to date. All too often I hear of teachers being asked to teach something outside of their scope of certification, just because it is easier than hiring a new instructor. Remaining certified is expensive because instructors must attend yearly educational events to learn the latest research and newest safety protocols.

Pretending to be qualified to yoga, weightlifting, Zumba, or Essentrics® for example, not only puts students at risk but this kind of behaviour can invalidate an instructor's insurance. Just because you as a teacher are certified to deliver one type of fitness class, does not then mean that you can use your own 'smarts' to fake it through teaching another discipline. If this becomes the norm then where will we be years from now?

Potential customers want the least expensive, best fitness experience that they can find but the hard truth is, education is expensive and qualified staff need to be paid well to offset the cost of maintaining their credentials. We need to be responsible consumers and demand only the best or teachers will stop spending the money necessary to keep up to date and then the health and safety of clients is put at risk.

I used to lead aqua fitness classes at a facility near my home. I had all of the proper qualifications. My boss asked the lifeguard to write down my choreography while I was teaching. He then called me that night and fired me, saying that he could pay her half of what he was paying me and therefore didn't need me anymore. While someone can go to YouTube university or pretend to know what they are doing for a certain amount of time, the lack of education will eventually become apparent. You want to make sure that when it comes to your health, your fitness professionals and physicians and physiotherapist have the proper training and licences.

My advice: if your gym is super cheap, just make sure that the people training you are qualified and up to date in their certifications! I have worked at facilities where the trainers let their certifications fall out of date by ten and twenty years! We are always learning new ways to keep people safe and fit. Ask your trainer questions about their credentials. Your health is in their hands so you should demand only the best!

Beth

# THE BEST EXERCISE

February 22, 2016

In my business, I hear a lot said about "the best exercise."

While it is true that if you have an injury, or if you are physically limited in some way, there may be 'better' exercises for you to do than others, I believe that the best exercise is the one that you will actually do every day, or at least three times per week.

I love being in the gym and can be there for hours teaching or taking different classes. If someone said that the best exercise was cross country skiing or kick boxing and that nothing else can compare, I would be very discouraged, as I do not like either one of these activities. We are all motivated by different things and none of us will continue an activity that we do not like.

You have to find that one thing that you love so much, you will do it when the weather is unpleasant, or you are very busy. It is so easy to make excuses for not taking care of ourselves, that we need to tap into that one type of fitness that will keep us committed. Often we are our own worst enemy when it comes to commitment, so choose an activity that you enjoy and if you have not found it yet, keep looking.

Once you have found that perfect activity, you still need to train in a balanced way. Make sure that your whole body is being trained and not just the muscles used in the said activity. Find classes that will train for strength, balance and flexibility. You need to work on all the components of physical conditioning to remain injury free and able to participate fully in your favourite activity. For example, you might love tennis or pickle ball. To be able to keep doing this activity for years, you need to formally train to keep your muscles strong and flexible and you need to train your cardiovascular system as well. This might be the one thing that is missing in your routine because you do not like to formally workout but it is very important if you want to stay healthy and avoid overuse injuries from your favourite sport.

You have to keep your health in balance, to continue to live pain free, so while walking may be your favourite activity, your upper body muscles and core are atrophying if you are not training them. This fact can set you up for physical problems down the road which may take you away from walking.

Beth

# GET HEALTHY/FIT IN SIX MINUTES?

June 23, 2016

While browsing the books at Chapters yesterday, I was overwhelmed by the number of books promising 'quick fix' solutions to all manner of weight loss issues. What struck me is the focus on speed. Almost all diet or exercise books promise to help you achieve your goals within a very short time period. I've had many clients tell me that they have no time to exercise and these 'quick fix' books appeal to those people who want a fit body in the least amount of time possible.

The cold hard truth is there is no quick solution. Losing weight is hard and it takes commitment on many different levels that require time and energy. While a trainer can make a program for you that is condensed to fit your lifestyle, sustainable change involves alterations to your whole routine. The simple fact is you have to move more and eat less.

You must exercise and fuel your body with the proper foods that will satisfy your appetite and will give you energy to be active. You cannot expect to lose weight by exercising for just six minutes every morning, keep eating whatever you want and then sit for ten to twelve hours a day. I am not fond of book titles that make unrealistic promises, so be wary.

There is no magic pill that replaces exercise and proper eating. In my experience it's the clients who build their lives around their exercise routine, who have the most success. They select the classes that they want to attend or the physical activity that they will do every day and then they never let anything interrupt that commitment.

I have also found that the clients who join a gym have more success than the clients who try to do it on their own at home.

The only good thing about these books is that they encourage people to start thinking about their health. This is an important first step in weight loss and I hope that it will lead to seeking professional assistance. Often it is knowing that we have a gym to go to and that people are expecting to see us, that keeps us on track with our exercise goals.

Beth

# DON'T FORGET THE CARDIO

March 1, 2016

While it is important to work our muscles so that we can be functionally fit, it is also important to remember to work our heart! Balanced training is the key to good health. For example, I had not seen a particular client of mine for a few months when suddenly we had the chance to work together again for a brief period of time. This gentleman is in his mid-sixties and he is one of the strongest men I know. He works hard at the gym, constantly working to keep himself in good shape.

When I changed up the programming to add eight minutes of light jogging at the beginning of the class, I was shocked to see that he was completely out of breath after five minutes. A year ago, he used to be able to jog for far longer. It became clear to me that he has stopped working on the cardio component of his fitness regime. Sometimes we only do what we like to do at the gym. Perhaps it is what we find easiest. This can be a real mistake. That is why I often remind my clients, as they moan and groan, that I am not there to be their friend but to help them work through all of the components of fitness so that they work out in a balanced manner.

Many of my students are using fitness trackers as they try to walk a certain number of steps everyday. While you are walking, try to include some interval training into your pace. Try walking at a faster pace for fifteen seconds to two minutes, and then drop down to your normal pace for a period of time and repeat as you feel that you can handle it. In time you will improve your aerobic power.

My message today is to stay in tune with your overall health. Most of my students are strong and flexible. Just make certain that you can go the distance as well.

# INTERVAL TRAINING: IS IT FOR YOU?

May 17, 2016

While on my way to work yesterday, I heard a Montreal doctor talking on a local radio show about interval training. The discussion was about whether working harder for shorter intervals is better than working at a moderate intensity for a longer period of time.

I decided to weigh in on the issue because I have had some questions regarding this type of training from my students. A few would like to see it offered at our gym. For the record, I work with clients whose average age is 68 years old. My students are very fit.

Interval training involves working as hard as you can for two minutes (the timed intervals vary) and then recovering for a short period of time before giving it your all again. The key to achieving any benefit from this type of training is your ability to give each interval your best effort. It is an excellent way to improve the cardio component of your workout.

The question is, is it for you?

If you have a heart condition it can be dangerous to push yourself to your absolute limit. You have to tell your doctor what you want to do and get clearance ahead of time. Pushing people to their limit involves risk. My advice is to make sure that you are in good physical condition beforehand and if it gets to be too hard, lower the intensity by walking on the spot.

If you have joint issues such as bad knees, back, shoulder or neck, my primary concern with interval training is that you must be mindful of your posture throughout the workout. Often when we are training fast, our posture begins to get sloppy and we can get injured easily. Keep the intervals simple, safe, and watch your posture as you begin to tire.

I hesitate to call interval training the best exercise because in my opinion the best training for you, is the one that you enjoy and the one that will get you to the gym regularly. Some people hate interval training so even if it was the best exercise, they would not do it, but they would walk on a treadmill or lift weights.

There is no quick fix, perfect exercise or diet. If you want do interval training attend a reputable class, with a qualified instructor, or hire a trainer to work with you privately on intervals that are safe for you. The key to an effective workout regime is variety, so adding interval training is a great way to break out of your routine. If you want to add intervals of varying speed to your workout you must be mindful of maintaining correct posture throughout because it may compound problems that you already have with your knees and/or back.

The great thing about joining a fitness facility is that you can try a variety of classes to find your own favourite way to burn calories.

Keep safe.

Beth

# REIKI – WHAT IS IT AND HOW CAN I USE IT?

By Rob Cosh

November 22, 2020

Last week I was honoured to deliver presentation on the practice and application of Reiki to Beth's Virtual Fitness students. I am Master Teacher level Reiki practitioner in both the Usui and Holy Fire systems of Reiki. What follows is a brief overview of the main points from that presentation. Beth and I hope that this information gives you one more tool in your toolbox to help you meet the challenges we are facing today.

### What is Reiki?

Reiki is a holistic healing modality originating from Japan during the early 20th century. It was created by Mikao Usui. We refer to the original form of Reiki as Usui Reiki which is a holistic healing modality originating in Japan in early 19th century that contains elements of many esoteric healing practices. Recipients can expect to quickly reach a deep state of relaxation in which tension, stress and inflammation begin to drop, allowing Chi energy to circulate more easily through the body.

### What is Reiki Doing?

Reiki is known to activate the parasympathetic nervous system. This is associated with lower heart rate, lower blood pressure and improved heart rate variability. It has been linked with lower cortisol production. Cortisol is known as the "stress hormone." All of these "bio-markers" are linked with many prevalent chronic illnesses. Of course, it stands to reason that if we could improve these physiological markers, there would be tangible health benefits!

### The Woo-Woo Stuff

Reiki is a form of spiritual practice. Spiritual, but not religious. It is not dogmatic. It does not require belief or faith of any kind. It is energy-based and is not in conflict with any known religion. Consider that across millennia and in cultures throughout the world, the laying on of hands is a shared approach to healing and comfort. Makes you think, doesn't it? This form of healing is innate in humans and is easily learned or uncovered – anyone can do this.

### If Reiki is Real, Why is There No Proof?

This is a very common question, and understandably so. We live in a world of instant gratification, and all of civilization's knowledge is searchable at any time it seems. We've become accustomed to the capitalization of science – insofar as scientific research seems to be largely related to endeavours to find saleable products and technologies. It's hard to envision a pharmaceutical company funding research into an innate healing ability that is easily learned and used without the need for any additional materials.

It's important to realize that although we are conditioned to look for proof, the common drug Aspirin was used for 70 years before science understood why it worked! Science is, in fact, constantly re-writing itself as new knowledge is discovered. The world was flat for centuries, until we realized it wasn't. It is interesting to note, however, that Reiki is being used officially in over 700 hospitals in the USA (2014 data). Science may not understand Reiki, yet – but it accepts that improved patient outcomes, reduced hospital stays and drug costs are associated with the practice of Reiki and welcomes the practice into their operations.

### Reiki Will Not....

- Mend your broken bones.
- Cure your diseases.
- Bring you money or fame.

- Do any miraculous thing you may have heard.

**However, Reiki Will....**

- Give your physical and energetic/emotional body a calming experience, and when we are still, our innate healing processes can take place.

- Our bodies are immensely sophisticated and can produce all of the compounds we need to heal if we provide the right inputs. (nutrition/exercise/mental health/energetic health)

- Create a sense of openness and connectedness, often resulting in a reduction of mental fog, fatigue, clarity in decision making, improved mood and demeanor.

- Attract your pets.

One of the greatest aspects of Reiki is that the benefit is gifted to both the receiver AND the practitioner. If you become certified to practice Level 1 Reiki, or beyond, you will receive every Reiki treatment that you give to another. It's so efficient! It's also the most relaxing way to spend an hour here or there. There aren't many things more wholesome than being in service to another.

**Reiki During COVID**

Reiki can provide ourselves with another "good" input towards a balanced, less inflamed system of health, along with exercise and nutrition. Universal to indigenous healing systems around the world are working to help create systemic balance for the recipient. Reiki supports this directly. In these harried and harrowing times, Reiki can help restore calm and reduce anxiety – directly impacting the physiology of stress, which can help reduce inflammation, improve cardiovascular health and move us closer to a state of relaxation – where our bodies can most effectively do the physical healing that we need.

I encourage you to explore Reiki by seeking out a local practitioner you feel an affinity with and arranging to have a Reiki session.

**Rob Cosh / Master Teacher / Usui and Holy Fire Reiki Systems**

# THE MAGIC OF 20

January 29, 2020

People often tell me that they admire my ability to complete projects and then they go on to tell me why they could never do what I have done. I hear excuses like, "I can't find the time" or "the job is too big."

I have managed to achieve my goals because I embraced the magic of 20 and used it in both my writing and in my fitness classes and the results are impressive. I am here to tell you that you can be successful as well. Whether you are trying to lose weight through exercise or write your memoir, just break the task down into timed bits and before you know it, you will have something to celebrate!

I started teaching Tabata last year, which is a type of training that demands students do a challenging fitness move for only twenty seconds followed by ten seconds of rest. We complete eight cycles and then take one minute to rest before starting another round. My students are improving their cardiovascular fitness through this simple concept of doing little spurts of energy for short periods of time.

The truth is you have to work hard to improve your cardiovascular fitness level and most people don't have the time to work out for hours on end to achieve great results. Tabata allows for an increase in cardiovascular stamina without the need for many long hours of traditional aerobic exercise. My class is packed with students. People love this simple and yet effective way of getting into better shape.

How do I use the magic of 20 in my writing? In 2016, I started writing in twenty minute increments followed by a mandatory five minute break, and this has resulted in three published books!

I'm currently writing four books and in order to get them done, I work on each of them for only twenty minutes a day. I get up at five am so that I can write for two hours before I have to get ready for my busy day of teaching, but if early morning doesn't appeal to you, maybe you can carve out twenty minutes in the evening. The important thing is to find the time that suits you best and then set your timer.

This magic of 20 eliminated my procrastination habit. I could no longer say that I had no time to devote to writing a book. Everyone can find twenty minutes in their day for any activity. Set a timer and stop working after it rings. Do this daily and before you know it you will have achieved your goal.

The answer is simple but for some reason we make it complicated. Get busy!

Beth

# TABATA TRAINING

February 20, 2019

If you attend the gym where I work, you have noticed that I have added a new class. Next session it will be called Tabata Tuesday. It is a version of interval training or high intensity interval training (HIIT), where we work as hard as we can for twenty seconds and then take ten seconds to rest, and we repeat this cycle for eight rounds. After each round, we walk it off and rest for thirty seconds to one minute before we begin the protocol again. This gives our body a chance to recover. Each round lasts about four to five minutes and we do this for twenty to twenty-five minutes. We then do some standard muscle conditioning and stretching to complete the hour.

If you were attending my Aerobic Interval class for the last year, you know that I have been doing this type of training for quite awhile, but the intervals were longer. Tabata rounds are more intense by design i.e., jumping jacks or jogging with high knees, as most of us can push ourselves to do something challenging for twenty seconds. This type of training is a great way to safely push ourselves out of our comfort zone. I always offer a low impact option to the high impact exercises so everyone can participate.

When we attend the same classes all the time we can suffer from a condition where our body has adapted, and we stop seeing improvements in our fitness. Adding this type of class to your weekly workout regime is a great way to shake up your system. Sherri told me last week that she felt she had so much energy after our Tabata workout that she was 'bouncing' through the rest of her day. I was so happy to hear this.

Tabata is named after Dr. Izumi Tabata who studied two groups of exercisers in 1996. One group worked at a moderate intensity for one hour, five days a week for six weeks, the other trained at high intensity for short periods of time with rest periods in between. The results were impressive enough that interval training became a huge part of the fitness industry. You can do your own research on the amazing benefits from training in this fashion. Google will lead you to lots of great articles.

As Len Kravitz, Ph.D., explains in his article published in the June 2018 issue of canfitpro magazine, *Why Less is More,* "the higher your Vo2 max, the greater cardio protection you have from cardiovascular disease" (Kravitz. pg.29). When we train at our upper limit (Vo2 max) for short periods of time we are attempting to improve the functioning of our cardiorespiratory system. We work hard at the gym to gain strength and flexibility, but we also want to challenge our heart to keep it in top shape. Since this is heart health month, let's give a bit of love to our hard-working hearts and try this new workout.

Beth

# AEROBICS HAS A BAD NAME

January 2021

What is on my mind today is the lack of love for good old-fashioned aerobics. Even though I still teach it to my students, I am here to tell you that it has become a thing of the past.

Now that I am training future teachers, I see how much the industry has changed based on the interests of my canfitpro students. While I have been busy creating successful fitness classes and working my butt off to deliver them well, the industry has evolved to the point where young people hear the word 'aerobics' and they run for the hills. I have yet to meet a candidate who wants to put in the time to master the 32-count phrase and patterning. Really any exercise that gets your heart rate up and keeps it up is aerobic but the next generation want to teach interval classes or bootcamp and not v-steps and grapevines.

I love learning new skills and being able to offer variety to my students. I am sad that today's teachers are not interested in exploring some of the 'old' ways but now I sound like an old lady. I am always taking new courses and expanding my teaching capabilities. What is old will become new again once people tire of doing jumping jacks and burpees.

Now back to my grapevines!

Beth

# CANADIANS GET FAILING GRADE ON FITNESS

October 29, 2019

Participaction, a non-profit group promoting healthy living, recently released a study that gives Canadians a 'D' for overall physical activity. Simply put, we are spending too much time sitting in front of our screens which can lead to weight gain, disease, and physical atrophy. This information makes me sad because my whole life is centered around trying to get people moving. While my classes are full and my students are fit, the challenge is getting newcomers into the gym. I even became a PRO TRAINER with canfitpro to train tomorrow's fitness leaders to help with this challenge.

We should be getting a minimum of 150 minutes of exercise each week or approximately 20 minutes each day but very few people are achieving this, and I can't understand why. Some people need a 'white coat' or doctor to tell them that their very life depends on getting more active, while others need an injury of some kind, perhaps to their back or knee, to drive them to change their behavior. Here are some simple ways to build more activity into your day.

First and foremost, try to stand more if you have a desk job. Many employers will give you a standing desk. If this is not an option, try to stand up and shake out the legs often during the day. In fact, stand up right now. You can feel the blood move down into the legs and right away that improves your circulation. Get out for a walk on your lunch break. Even just 10 to 15 minutes would help. Park far away from the entrances to stores.

You can find affordable treadmills second-hand that can fold up and store away easily. We purchased a demo model treadmill about 12 years ago. We spent a fair amount of money on it but it was worth every penny.

I find it easiest to dress in my fitness clothes, right out of bed. Get up a bit earlier, put on your gear and walk on your treadmill or outside for a few minutes. You will have so much more energy if you begin the day with a good heart pumping sweat. Put your treadmill in your living room. I mean it. If you see it, you are more likely to use it.

Ask a friend to become an exercise buddy. Honestly, the people who train together, keep each other accountable. While it is easy to avoid a workout when we are alone, very few of us would let down a friend.

Get yourself a dog! Of course, you have to have the time and resources for this, but I know of at least two people who changed their health in a positive way because they got themselves a rescue dog. The pets forced them to go for long walks several times a day and in the process, they reversed disease.

I sound like broken record because I talk so much about the benefits of exercise. I just want people to know that the secret to good health is in their hands.

Studies like this tell me that my job is not done. I need to try to reach more people with this message.

I hope to see you in my classes soon and bring a friend!

Beth

# POLE DANCING: WHAT A WORKOUT!

September 29, 2016

Yes, I tried pole dancing and it had absolutely nothing to do with sex and everything to do with physical strength! My daughter who has been participating in this pole dancing for years was allowed to bring a guest on the last day of her fitness session. We were invited to try or simply watch. I figured I would just sit on the side and observe but curiosity got the best of me.

Would I be able to get myself up on the pole and would I be able to stay there? It was a safe learning environment and probably my only chance to answer these questions, so I gave it a whirl. I learned very quickly that it requires a tremendous amount of upper body and abdominal strength to do this workout. I currently teach 16 hours of fitness a week and I found it incredibly challenging and humbling.

I was not a fan of spinning around the pole. Perhaps this gets easier with time. I appreciate the physical stamina needed to do an hour of this class, and if it encourages my daughter to get stronger and more fit in the process, I am happy for her and everyone else who is brave enough to take this class. The best exercise is the one that you will actually do!

At some point the girls were in handstands beside the pole using it for balance. When was the last time you tried doing a handstand or climbing a rope or tree? It certainly appeals to the kid in all of us. This workout is a great way to laugh and lighten up and get fit all at the same time.

Beth

# YOUR GYM CAN BE ANYWHERE

September 4, 2017

I am quite lucky that I have a husband who supported me and my career by turning our whole basement into a gym. I take it for granted and assume that everyone has a space dedicated to fitness in their homes but the truth is you don't need a fancy space to get fit.

I recommend however that whatever area you do have be ready and welcoming. You are far more likely to exercise on days when you cannot get to the gym, if you have a small area of your home that you can clear quickly and easily enough to set up a yoga mat. As a personal trainer, I have seen the spaces that work best and well, the ones that need some improving.

Most often the treadmill in any home is covered with clothes or folded up and tucked away so tightly that getting it out to use would be the exercise itself. Usually, the equipment is in the basement which is dark, cluttered and secluded so no one ever goes down there to use it, or the weights that are collecting dust in the corner.

The fall season brings about cooler weather so why not spend some time today preparing for those days when you are less likely to get to class. Look at your space and set up a dedicated area for mat work. It doesn't have to be big or impressive. It need only be ready for you when you cannot get to the gym.

Beth

# #1 FITNESS TREND IN CANADA

December 19, 2018

Every year canfitpro, Canada's fitness education leader, takes a survey of its professionals across Canada to determine the most popular trend. For the second year in a row, Functional Fitness has topped the chart. I am excited to see this as I began to introduce this concept into my classes years ago and it is the reason that I wrote my book, *Fundamental Fitness After Fifty – Three at Home Fitness Programs to Keep You Functionally Fit for Life.* https://www.betholdfield.ca/product-page/fundamental-fitness-over-fifty

Perhaps because I grew up with older parents and watched them struggle with low mobility when they were in their mid-seventies, I decided that I needed to help my students avoid this as much as possible. Many of my students began attending my classes when they retired in their late fifties or early sixties and they continue with me today, almost 20 years later. I build my programs based on the idea that we want to be able to move in a functional way, so the exercises that we do in class mimic movements that are needed to perform activities of daily living and those used in popular sports.

I work hard to create programs that keep my students interested, challenged and injury free. I am always looking for ways to improve their performance in their favourite sports so we train for many of the movements that are common in golf, hockey, curling, skiing, and racket sports. It is important to me that my clients be able to move about their day with ease.

The second most popular trend in fitness was HIIT and the third trend was Older Adult Training. Baby Boomers are looking for ways to stay active. Based on this survey, it would appear that I am on the right path and my students are too!

# THE BENEFITS OF LINE DANCE

January 31, 2018

Line Dance has a bad rap. If you've never tried it, chances are the first thing that comes to your mind is country music; cowboy boots and wedding receptions, where people goof around on the dance floor after a few drinks. While it is that, it is also a serious medium for improving fitness. I know this because I have been leading dance classes to many of the same students since 2011.

I can honestly tell you that I have never had so much fun while improving my memory, coordination, balance and cardiovascular health as I do in my dance classes. We laugh together when we make mistakes and cheer with joy when we get through some of the more complicated dances without error. The social bonding is second to none. Students hate to miss their dance lesson not just because of the new steps being showcased but for the camaraderie that the class provides.

There have been many reports circulating around the internet as of late touting the benefits of dance. From my perspective, I have witnessed a drastic improvement in cognitive function, co-ordination and balance in all of my line dance students. While it may have been hard to remember 16 counts of steps a few years ago, it is much easier to master the 48- and 64-count dances today. The ability to remember complicated footwork after hearing just a few bars of a familiar song is incredible. And the ability to process the new information quickly is astounding.

Music lifts our mood and motivates us to succeed and when we dance along to our favourite song, we feel invincible. There really is no better feeling! With each success our confidence grows and I have seen this new found determination work its way into other aspects of my students' lives. We are more eager to try new tasks when we feel confident and capable.

Learning new things will keep you young.

Find a class and get dancing today. Even if it is difficult at first, you will eventually succeed and find joy! I promise.

Beth

# WHY YOGA?

August 14, 2015

This week I came across three people in my life who expressed their dislike for yoga. In two of the cases the individuals said that they hate moving so slowly. In the third case, the person said that it makes her nauseous. I have one client who did not want to be in my yoga class because she felt it was some sort of cult and that it would go against her religion.

There are several reasons why people dislike yoga. One thing that yoga does is it forces us to slow down and face our limitations both emotional and physical. Many people hate being alone with their thoughts. In my classes, we usually hold the poses/stretches for five deep breaths. Learning to relax into the pose and accept what it is teaching you about your body and mind is challenging and therefore not for everyone.

My first experience with yoga was 'Hot Yoga.' I took a friend of mine. The room was very hot and we were doing extremely challenging poses in that heat for 90 minutes. My friend threw up and passed out! I hated the experience, especially since I had told the teacher that it was my first class and then after telling me to go at my own pace, he chastised me anytime I came out of the pose to take a break! I am happy to say that I did go to another yoga class and it was there that I found peace and relaxation.

My message today is there are many different styles of yoga and many interesting classes, so if you have had a bad experience in one, try another. I am not a perfect yogi by any stretch of the imagination, but I do my best to show people the benefits of regular yoga practice.

In my fitness classes I have been incorporating yoga postures for years during the stretching component, but without using yoga terms. For those athletes who do not want to be caught doing yoga, I would speak about the balance challenge and for those wanting the stretch, I would focus on teaching them how the pose is helping to keep them flexible.

The key is simply to get moving. Once people start to feel their bodies in ways that are unknown to them, the benefits start to unfold. Now my clients actually ask me for more 'yoga stretching.' Yesterday, after I had taught fitness for a few hours my body was not happy. My right hip was in pain and it was radiating to my lower back. I immediately went into my stretches from my physiotherapist, which also happen to be common yoga postures and I found relief.

Find a friend and go to a new yoga class this weekend. You will laugh together and maybe in the process you will reap some benefits for your body and mind.

Beth

# FITNESS TRACKER CONCERN

May 31, 2017

While on my way to work yesterday morning I heard an interview with Dr. Mitch Shulman on CJAD. Dr. Mitch was stating his concern that though fitness trackers are great for motivating us to exercise often, we need to be careful if we are using the calorie counting component of this popular gadget.

The fitness trackers are meant to be used by the general population and they are not necessarily calibrated specifically to your body type. For instance, someone who is heavier may burn more calories while walking the same distance as someone who is lighter, simply because they are carrying more weight over the same distance and time period. The danger lies in us thinking that if we have burned x amount of calories in our exercise session, we can have that second piece of dessert and not gain any weight. This may indeed be false and result in unwanted weight gain.

It is better to discuss your calorie needs with a registered nutritionist to know exactly how many calories you need to consume, and how many you need to lose, in order to achieve your specific fitness goals.

In my opinion, no machine can replace personalized, professional service. Know the limits of your tracker and use it wisely, and always seek the advice of trained professionals.

Beth

# ENERGY BOOSTING WORKOUT

November 28, 2018

One of my students came up to me last week to inform me that she has a bounce in her step since she started taking my Essentrics® classes last year. This woman is in her early sixties and leads an active life. She is still working part time and attending the gym a few times per week when she can. I have heard this quite a bit since I began teaching this technique in October of 2017. I had just finished reading about the positive impact that Essentrics® has on the cardio-respiratory system when she spoke to me, so I was happy to let my student know why she was feeling this way.

In the workouts we regularly contract and then relax our muscles, which promotes blood flow around the body. We also move within our stretches instead of simply holding still, and we rotate within and around all of the joints which brings new blood into stiff areas, promoting rejuvenation. More blood means more oxygen is being delivered and this coupled with the fact that we are unlocking stiff joints, adds to the feeling of increased energy at the end of each class. Because we are constantly pulling up in our posture, we breathe better as well. All of this puts a spring in our step as we move about our day.

I love it when you share your success stories with me as I can pass them on and hopefully motivate someone to try a class for themselves.

Beth

# SHOULD YOU TRY ESSENTRICS®?

November 20, 2017

I have been asked this question by some of my students recently because I will be teaching Essentrics® in January in Pointe Claire and many of my long time students are wondering if they should give this workout a try. The answer is, yes! I always recommend trying different forms of fitness because you might find that the new approach suits you better than the classes that you have been attending for years.

For example, I know of two students who were very upset because they had to give up my Step class years ago because of arthritis. They tried water aerobics and discovered that it was far less painful on their hips and knees. They were pleasantly surprised by the experience and never felt the need to return to their old training ground. Trying new classes challenges our minds as well as our muscles which is good for the body as a whole.

An Essentrics® workout is very different from my standard cardio/muscle classes. Though the music will be motivating, it is not the same type of environment because the tempo is slower. We usually perform the class in bare feet which is recommended. Our feet are so restricted in our shoes that we have inadvertently caused imbalances that travel right up through the legs into our backs. Being barefoot allows us to correct these imbalances. If you insist on wearing your shoes just pay special attention to movements that might affect your knee such as side to side lunges.

We are moving slower than in my standard classes which gives you time to focus on your posture. The movements are designed to simultaneously stretch and strengthen the muscles and re-balance the whole body. Though we are not lifting weights, we work just as hard because the body is working against gravity, eccentrically. You will leave the class feeling energized, taller and refreshed instead of 'beat up.'

If you sit tall right now you will see how much harder it is to maintain proper posture. Roll the shoulders back and down. Open the chest and pull up through your abdominal wall. Most people can hold this position for a short time but before long, the majority of us will start to slouch down again because it is easier. In Essentrics® we maintain this erect posture through-out the class and then add movements that target hard to reach muscles in our back, abdominals, legs and arms. The focus is on being 'pulled up' at all times, reaching and extend-ing our body toward the ceiling. We then move slowly in all directions and end up exercising muscles that have not been used in a long time. You are familiar with the old adage, 'if you don't use it, you will lose it.' An Essentrics® workout exercises every muscle in the body which promotes cell regeneration and rejuvenation.

Remember that it is still a workout. The first time that you try the class you will feel muscles that you have not felt in awhile. You may experience some mild discomfort the next day or during the class but I can tell you that it feels so good after-ward, you will want to return. I have been doing this workout since the end of September and I already see a difference in my body. My midsection has slimmed down and the stretching has helped to re-balance my body, which has alleviated pain in my neck, shoulders and back.

So yes, you should give Essentrics® a try if you can. If you cannot find a class in your area you can go to essentrics.com and order DVDs to do at home.

Beth

# 8 HOURS OF SILENCE?

November 25, 2016

Many of you know that today I was supposed to be attending a silent retreat in Ottawa. Unfortunately, the event was cancelled yesterday afternoon but I thought I would take a moment to address the 'how' and 'why' of one of these retreats.

A number of you mentioned to me that you would never be able to be in a group of people and be completely silent for that many hours. In fact some of you suggested that it would be impossible to be quiet for longer than an hour. I have attended several of these experiences and what they have taught me is how easy it actually is, and how much I long for longer periods of silence.

The first time you go into silence is a bit daunting but you must remember that you are being guided the whole time by the teacher in the room. If you have attended yoga classes, it is like this but simply longer. We usually begin with meditation which is guided and it sets the theme for the day. One of the retreats was about forgiveness, another about self care. I have been to about six and each has its own purpose.

After meditation we do yoga and then have a morning snack. All of the food is raw and meant to sustain you in your day long practice. In the past, we have done art, journaling and walking meditation. We are often put into restorative yoga poses designed to release tension in the body.

The idea is to have a place where we can actually hear ourselves think. There is meditation music playing softly in the background but there is no Internet access and there are no other voices in the room except that of the teacher. It is referred to as a 'safe space' where we can let go and listen to our own hearts and thoughts.

By the end you feel like you have been on a week long vacation. It is amazing how much we are bombarded by noise and images all day long. We only realize how exhausting this is on our nervous system when we take the time to remove the constant buzz from our day.

I hope that you get a chance to participate in one of these retreats. It is a challenge at first but once you try it, it becomes something that you crave. Silence really is golden.

Beth

# THE IMPORTANCE OF FLEXIBILITY TRAINING

February 1, 2016

Today's post is directed primarily at those who come to the gym regularly to train on their own in the weight room. These individuals are serious about their fitness regime, but I am sad to say that most of them spend too much time training the same muscles in exactly the same way and practically no time stretching to improve their flexibility. It is so important to train all of your muscles in a balanced way.

For example, you should not train your abdominals, without also training your back. You should not just train your biceps and forget about your triceps. If you do neglect to train the opposing muscle group, you can end up being out of balance and could cause yourself injury.

In addition, if you train your muscles to be strong, you must also train them to be flexible. If we do not do this, our range of motion may be limited, which puts us at risk for tearing a tendon or a muscle. Simple movements like bending over to pick something up, or twisting quickly to catch a ball, can result in strains and tears if we are not flexible. If you have ever been to a physiotherapist, you know that they often identify the tight muscle group as part of the problem, if not the main cause of the injury.

About five years into my career, I added fifteen minutes of stretching at the end of every one of my fitness classes because I knew that outside of yoga class, regular fitness students needed to spend more time improving their flexibility to remain healthy and pain free. If you go to betholdfield.ca stretching videos that contain the important stretches you should be doing daily.

Please start to add a minimum of five to ten minutes of stretching to your exercise regime.

Beth

# BENEFITS OF GROUP FITNESS

March 27, 2019

Last summer I had the pleasure of leading my extended family through a yoga class by the water, up at the cottage. What is on my mind today are the many benefits associated with group exercise.

When we join a gym and participate in the Group X classes:

1. We get a chance to compare our fitness levels with people our own age or those who may be older or younger. This can be a bit of wake up call for some that more exercise is needed but it can also encourage us if we are able to keep up!

2. So much laughter takes place in my classes. I'm sure that some of us may go through the day and never have the opportunity to smile, much less belly laugh, especially if we are always alone. Laughing with others feels good and this social connection lifts our spirits, making the experience of exercise enjoyable. This keeps us coming back which is good for our health!

3. The students form bonds that continue outside of the gym and they begin to share and care for each other which has a positive effect on health and fitness all around. We want to know why our friends are missing and we reach out to them to offer support!

4. We learn by watching others with physical limitations that anything is possible. Sometimes we can get discouraged by our own aches and pains but when we get together and witness our classmates overcome their challenges it is incredibly motivating!

5. In group classes, even though we can participate at our own level by making the movements easier, we are mov-

ing through the experience as one unit, lifting each other up along the way with our smiles, high fives, whoops and hollers of joy or groans of pain.

I can't help but smile when I am teaching my classes because I get so much joy from watching all of this go on during our time together. Yes, it can be rewarding to go for a good run or walk alone but nothing compares to the positive energy and benefits of participating in Group X. If you have yet to try a class, what are you waiting for?

See you soon,

Beth

# PART TWO

# FITNESS TIPS AND TRICKS

**M**y nephew, Rob, who happens to be only five years younger than me, said something to me fifteen years into my career that shaped my perspective forevermore. During one of our family dinners, we were sequestered in the corner of the living room indulging in philosophies about life, sipping our coffees and talking about our respective careers. I expressed some doubt as to whether I was knowledgeable enough about my profession to which he said, "Beth, someone who has been doing a job like yourself for close to twenty years, IS THE EXPERT. That is literally the definition of what it means to be at the top of your game!"

His words took me by surprise. I had never considered myself to be an expert because I was too young. Sure, I had my little fitness job that I went to each day where my classes were packed with happy customers. My clients were seeing results because of the programs that I designed each month and that is why they were returning but I just thought that this was normal. I was simply doing a good job, at my job, but Rob helped me to see the huge impact that my class designs were having on the 50+ crowd. I needed someone to point out to me the unique quality that makes me stand out from the rest. I genuinely care about the wellbeing of my clients. I am not simply collecting a paycheck. While I still shy away from the concept of expert, I started my blog to give my experienced opinion about all topics related to fitness so that my students could remain injury free and healthy.

In the following section I offer tips and tricks to inspire you to keep moving even when life gets challenging. Enjoy!

# FIND YOUR MOTIVATION

November 9, 2015

As I move about my day, I see many people who need to exercise. I see young people who are carrying a dangerous amount of excess weight. I see middle aged people who have let themselves go for whatever reason and are now complaining of sore knees and backs. I come across seniors who think that golfing, curling and walking is all that they need to do to be fit.

Unless I am approached, I keep my thoughts to myself but I walk away with a lingering dread for these individuals. There is no "free pass," people. If you have no symptoms of disease or degeneration yet, that is great news but chances are there is something building if you are overweight and inactive. You need to find your motivation to get into fitness and ward off the problems that all of us face eventually. You may be in formal exercise classes but still carrying excess weight. I am so happy that you are in class but perhaps you need to investigate your nutritional habits and see if there is something you can do to improve your health.

For instance, as a senior, life may be going along quite smoothly and then you may start experiencing falls for no apparent reason. (I heard of two serious falls from different students just last week). If your muscles and balance are weak when this stage hits, you may suffer greater consequences from falls. You may break bones or tear muscles or ligaments and those will take longer to heal if you are out of shape. All of the above will take you out of your routine and away from your favoured activities. Life changes in an instant and my policy has always been to make sure that my clients are prepared for these situations.

My point is do you really want to be the person whose story sounds something like this: "Well I ended up in the Emergency, I guess I should've been taking better care of myself!"

Should've. Would've. Could've. I hear it too often. The good news is that when I am hearing it, it usually means someone is joining my classes and starting to make a difference in their lives.

Find your motivation to make healthy habits before tragedy strikes.

Do not wait for your doctor to tell you that you need to get on medication to improve your health. Instead ask them if you are clear to start going to fitness classes!

Make a change today!

Beth

# MY TOP THREE TIPS FOR SUCCESS

May 4, 2015

The first truth you must accept is that simply walking and watching what you eat is not enough. While this is an important part of keeping fit, all of us need to be involved in weightlifting (building muscular capacity through resistance training) if we want to lose pounds and remain functional fit for life.

Please keep these three tips in mind when you are working with a certified trainer.

Tip#1: You Are the Boss of You

My students have heard me say this to them all of the time. You know your limits better than any trainer does. If it feels wrong or painful, stop. Walk away from any trainer who yells at you or does not listen to your concerns. There is a big difference between discomfort and pain. Quite often the trainer wants to impress you and therefore might not be fully listening.

Tip#2: Basic is Better

I have seen the fads come and go but my clients have stayed injury free for the last 15 years by doing the basic exercises safely. You do not need fancy equipment. To stay functional, you need to work your back, abdominals, legs, shoulders and arms and you need to stretch to stay flexible. You can do this all in your home with guidance or head to a reputable gym and hire a trainer to help you.

Tip#3: Be Patient and Give It a Chance

I learned a long time ago that if you are not having a good time, you will not be back! It takes time to find the right workout regime. Be patient with yourself. If you are new to a gym, give it two weeks to get to know people. Talk to the trainers and at least one other client so that you can begin to build connections that will keep you coming back on those days when staying home seems appealing. Your friends will get you out of bed!

Beth

# SMALL STEPS ARE KEY

April 19, 2015

I have heard many excuses for not exercising but one of the best came from someone I know quite well. "Well, if I have to exercise 15 hours a week like you do, I'm not even going to try!" In reality all it takes is the right attitude, a bit of discipline and you will be on your way to better health without having to move into your local gym and spend every waking hour working out.

Please don't try to change everything you are doing all at once. Small steps are the key to creating lasting changes in your health. I have seen clients fail because they tried to make up for lost time, by doing everything all at once. For example, eating only salad and participating in every single boot camp class that you can find, is going to leave you hungry, cranky, and miserable by the end of the week.

Find something physically active that you love to do, like dancing, golfing, yoga, swimming, and then simply commit to doing it a few times per week. Find a friend to do it with you. Schedule it in and commit to telling everyone you love that this is your time to take care of yourself.

Try to change one thing in your diet. Drinking more water. Eating less sugar. Cutting down on caffeine. In my experience, after two weeks of just moving more and making smarter food choices, you will start to feel awesome and then you will be ready for more changes.

Start small and celebrate your success. Above all else, try to have fun doing whatever you decide to do. Be fully present in whatever you are doing. Smile and relax. You are on your way to better health.

Beth

# NEVER SAY NEVER

February 6, 2020

After twenty years in the business, I have heard so many extreme views about different fitness trends that I know better than to panic about any one of them.

"Don't ever jump or lift both feet off of the ground! You will hurt your joints."

"Don't ever do the Plow yoga pose! It killed a lady once."

"Don't ever do sit-ups or full sit-ups! It will hurt your back."

"Don't lift ten pound free weights or you will look like a body builder."

"Don't exercise in bare feet, you will hurt yourself!"

I could go on and on...

The truth is all of the above items are accurate to a point, and that point depends on the individual performing the exercise. Perhaps you have been told by your physiotherapist to follow some of the above guidelines and in that case, I suggest you listen because the advice is tailored to your particular health situation. However many people like to take snippets of information and apply it to themselves without reason. And that is where we can have problems.

One size does not fit all when it comes to most areas in life and this includes fitness, so while I always listen to what the 'experts' are saying, I do my best to stay away from extremes because this is usually associated with panic. People don't want to experience pain or injury, so it is normal to follow the herd but I challenge you to always ask yourself "why?" Do your homework instead of listening to rhetoric.

As a trainer of teachers, I tell my students to evaluate the risk versus the benefit when they are designing their programs.

When it comes to group exercise, teachers want to stay on the safe side of the equation and not put people's health in jeopardy. That being said, if the teacher is hired to teach a group of elite athletes or sport enthusiasts to improve their performance, they might determine that certain exercises that are considered risky are exactly the right ones for their class.

We want easy fixes and solutions. "I will be fine and get exactly what I am looking for if I never do w or x and always do y and z!"

If you have been following my blog over the last five years, I have reminded you that the only constant is change and the best kind of exercise is the one that is varied. Doing the exact same exercises for years is not necessarily safer because of overuse injuries and the potential for muscular imbalances to occur. Variety is the spice and key to life!

When you hear extreme fitness advice, do your homework. Look for the source, listen to the experts and then decide what is right for you based on your health situation which might mean seeking the advice of a qualified trainer.

Beth

# PUT YOURSELF FIRST

April 21, 2015

I see it all the time. Loving, caring folks, who give up their established fitness routines to help a loved one who is in need. While we must help those around us in challenging times, what worries me is when students let trivial things get in the way of making to class. The truth is once we start missing workouts, it gets easier and easier to make everything else a priority. Today I am telling you to put yourself first!

Set your exercise time and stick to it. If you are deeply committed to getting healthier, you must find a time in the day when "things" will not get in the way. I now have students who understand this and make their routines around class, no exceptions. I even have a student who is job searching and is only considering jobs that match her fitness class schedule. Now that is a bit extreme, but I am so happy to see that she is committed to staying healthy because once you miss one class or one session, it is easy to miss the next and then the next.

Caring for others is what you do but you need to care for yourself first so you can take care of the ones you love. We must keep our knees and backs and shoulders and mind etc., in good shape.

Everyone can get up a bit earlier. Set the alarm. Go for a walk before everyone else in the house gets up or exercise to an exercise video. Do it for the ones you love, if you will not do it for yourself!

Beth

# "REMEMBER WHY YOU STARTED"

August 13, 2015

Last month I watched Joss Stone, an English soul singer and songwriter, being interviewed on a Canadian entertainment show. The interviewer asked her how she handles criticism. She went on to talk about how hard it can be to be judged but that she believes the key is to "remember why you started."

To me this quote has great meaning. It is so easy to be dragged down by criticism in the fitness industry as we are constantly having to measure ourselves up against the latest, coolest trend. Some of the things I see make me question what my place will be in the future when I have no interest in hanging from ropes to do yoga or trampoline workouts.

If I remember why I started, it is because I love teaching. I love helping people be the best that they can be. I want my students to come to my classes feeling like they will be safe and cared for properly. I want them to know that I consider myself to be a partner in their efforts to get healthier. Together with their doctor's care and perhaps a physiotherapist's advice, I hope to help my students enjoy a pain free experience that makes them fall in love with exercise.

I believe in doing the basics better. I believe in working out in a balanced fashion. I try very hard to not to swing to the extremes in anything I do, as in my opinion that is where injuries occur.

I remember that as a little girl, my favourite thing to do was pretend I was the teacher! I love sharing my passion for dance and fitness with my students.

This is why I started! To spread the passion.

Beth

# "THE HIGH COST OF LOW LIVING"

October 25, 2016

I heard this expression yesterday on a talk show and it stuck with me. The discussion was about the upcoming changes to Canada's food guide and food labeling. The government is hoping that the changes will better inform people about healthy eating. A nurse called up to say that she is happy with these changes because of the "high cost of low living."

Processed foods are cheaper than fresh fruit and vegetables and this nurse was warning people that eating cheap foods comes with a high price to our health. Too much sugar, salt, and unhealthy fat, leads to obesity, diabetes and heart disease. I would add that refusing to invest in your health by joining a gym or hiring a personal trainer comes at a high cost as well. It's not just about the food you eat.

Yes, programs can be expensive but avoiding formal exercise altogether can have a negative impact on your health down the road. To be honest, it is not usually cost that keeps people away from the gym. I rarely hear this as an excuse. It comes down to making better choices. One of my students has said to me for years that she prefers to pay for fitness classes, rather than medications ward off disease. Mariette sees fitness as a way say healthy.

Invest well in your health and save money and time later in life.

Beth

# DOES YOUR TRAINER CARE?

November 8, 2016

I have been a member of canfitpro since 2001 and have been collecting their magazines for many years. In going through them recently I started to see a trend among the editions. For the most part, it's evident to me that the basics of fitness have not changed very much over the years.

One of the prevalent messages throughout the issues is the need for trainers to listen well and show empathy for the students. For the most part, the writers are referring to private one-on-one training, but I believe that this is just as important when teaching group fitness classes.

As teachers we should be there to help our students achieve their goals. If students are not able to follow an exercise safely and effectively, I must adjust my cuing to meet their needs or abandon the exercise. Before I became a teacher, I can remember struggling to follow the choreography or the muscle conditioning component in some classes and being completely frustrated! This is not a good feeling and so I do my best to avoid creating an environment that is chaotic and demotivating. When clients come up to me with comments about a certain move or exercise, I listen and do my best to adjust the exercise if the concern is warranted.

Remember that my job is to take you out of your comfort zone safely so that you can continue to improve your health. If you always train in the same exact way, you are at risk for injury. Please always ask your trainer for alternatives if you feel the challenge is too great but do your best to try to the new exercises because your trainer has the bigger picture in mind when they are designing programs. Progressions are a necessary evil of fitness conditioning.

Beth

# POSTURE POWER AND EXERCISE

January 18, 2017

I'm guessing that most of you reading this post are sitting in a chair with your back rounded and your shoulders rolled forward. This usually means that your chin and your neck are out of alignment as well. I know this because I catch myself sitting like this all the time. I also know that you have just sat up taller and done a realignment because as soon as someone says the word 'posture' we all self adjust. I want you to try to remember to do this more often throughout your day.

Setting our posture is the first thing we do in my classes before we begin any weight training exercise, because if you exercise with bad posture not only do you reinforce it but over time you can get hurt. We want our body to be as strong as possible so when we need to lift something, we need to align all of the joints as best as possible to set ourselves up for success and it begins with posture.

So the next time you are in any class that requires lifting weights or even in your own home, do a body scan beforehand. Is your back straight? Are your shoulders rolled back and down as they should be? Is your neck aligned over your spine?

When people are new to the gym, they need to be reminded of this often and I can see a big difference in the clients who have been trained to do this posture check. Yes, we all slack off sometimes, but the key is to try to remember to keep "perfect" posture as much as possible. I use the term "perfect" very loosely here. Many of us have injuries that prevent us from obtaining perfect alignment but do what you can to keep yourself safe.

Remember that the body is a chain of mechanics and if one piece is not properly lined up, the chain is not as strong. Work on the weaknesses by seeking the help of a trainer or physiotherapist before they become a problem.

Are you sitting taller?

I thought so...we just need reminders. I used to send out emails to my clients reminding them to drink water...perhaps I need to start this again but for posture!

Beth

# WORKING OUT UNTIL YOU VOMIT?

January 15, 2016

I often hear ladies talking in the locker room about other classes that they are attending. As an instructor, I am always keen to know what students like about their classes, so it is interesting to be a fly on the wall and listen to these conversations.

I once overheard a few ladies expressing how hard the workout was that they had just completed. All of them looked completely exhausted and one lady said that she felt like vomiting! I just want all of my students to know that while I personally believe it is okay to have worked well, I hope that none of you feel that you have been pushed to the point of being sick to your stomach.

My mission in all of my classes is to keep people functionally fit. When you come out of a class you should feel like you have experienced a good sweat and perhaps some muscle fatigue but I hope that you do not feel so exhausted that you are done for the day! My hope is that you have more energy after the class. The next day, you may feel your muscles but I want you to tell me if they are so sore to the touch that you cannot move! As instructors, we want everyone to love our classes, so we are all are eager to know how to improve the experience of our students.

I have no desire to be the toughest teacher at our facility. Instead, I hope you feel noticed, cared for and challenged when you attend my classes. I am not there to beat you up or make you feel like you are not good enough. I am there to lift you up and keep you fit and strong while you are having fun.

Beth

# HOW TO SURVIVE JANUARY START-UP

January 5, 2020

It's normal to feel a bit stiff and sore if you haven't worked out because of the holidays. I myself didn't work out as much as I wanted to, so my body is rebelling by introducing new pains each day. The good news is that classes start back up again soon.

Remember to listen to your body if you've been on a fitness vacation for the last three weeks. Don't try to make up for all of the overeating and lack of movement on the first day back by pushing yourself too hard.

I've been teaching fitness since 1998 and every year I see the same explosion of clients into the gym the first week of January. People want to feel better but what ends up happening, particularly to new students, is they go too hard that first week and experience delayed onset of muscle soreness (DOMS) and think that they've hurt themselves or that fitness isn't for them and they never come back.

I hate losing new clients to this and it happens every January because of the fitness frenzy at the gym where classes are often packed to the maximum. Unfortunately, newcomers can slip through the cracks if they don't hear the importance of going at their own pace and if I don't get my message to them to hang in there for at least three classes because it gets easier if they do!

I want you to be successful achieving your fitness goals this winter so here are a few tips to help you to survive your first week back to classes.

1. Remember that you don't have to complete all of the repetitions of an exercise. Start slowly and build up gradually, particularly if you have been a couch potato for the last three weeks! This will result in less soreness the next day, which will make it easier for you to continue to train.

2. If you can, try to pick an Essentrics® class or a yoga class as your first workout. These classes are typically easier on the body and you are able to adapt the movements or take breaks without looking out of place.

3. Remember to build rest and recovery into your week. If you feel that you must attend most of the classes offered at the gym, be smart about your selections. For example, take a cardio/muscle conditioning class on Monday but take a stretching class the next day etc. If you work the same muscles in exactly the same way, each day, you will put yourself at risk for pain and injury. Variety is the key to keeping fit and healthy.

And my last tip: get a glass of water! I am 99% sure that you need it.

Beth

# ONE SIZE DOESN'T FIT ALL

January 9, 2019

Most of us have had bad experiences trying to wear "one size fits all" clothing and the same can be said for fitness. What works for you may not work for your friend at all! This is why I teach so many different types of classes and it is why I encourage all of my students to try new workouts. It is also why I discourage shopping for classes based on the time that they are offered, instead of what is best or safest for you personally. You shouldn't continue to beat yourself up in a class that is not suitable for your personal situation, simply because it is the only time you have to work out. Perhaps you are meant to try something new where you might find a better fit!

I love it when a client brings their best friend to their favourite class because friends who exercise together are more likely to succeed in achieving their goals. But it can be awkward if the guest struggles with the tempo of the class and feels out of place or even worse, gets hurt trying to keep up to their fit friend! I saw a bit of that this week in a few of my classes and I did my best to ease the situation by keeping things simple. I always say give a class at least three attempts before giving it up because I could be having a bad day or vice versa. After a few weeks though, it is okay to admit that the class does not suit you or fit your style.

We also shouldn't push our own workout style on our friends and family. It really is a personal choice. In one of my classes, a wife insists on bringing her husband and she spends the entire hour, pointing out what he is doing wrong. I believe that she means well but, in the end, she is cheating herself out of workout where she can let go and focus on herself.

The best thing I can do is encourage people to burn more calories than they are consuming by exercising every single day, in a way that hopefully pleases them. There is "no one size fits all" when it comes to both diet and fitness. Try new things but don't insist that your way is the best way or the only way to get in shape.

Beth

# COMMERCIALS AS YOUR FITNESS PROMPT

April 23, 2015

I am hoping that you have found a time in your day that you can devote to your health. For me, rising early fits well into my schedule but many people tell me that they have absolutely no free time. Try this...

In the evening, when you are watching TV, use the commercials as a prompt to move. Change what you are doing during each commercial and repeat for the duration of the time that you are watching television. Have some water nearby and a towel, just in case.

Commercial #1. Jog or march in place- hitting your hands with your knees.

Commercial #2. Five slow squats – Stand hip width apart, hip hinge forward as you send your bum back. Keep knees just in line with toes, not passed if possible. Lower to a pain free range or ninety degrees.

Commercial #3. Five Slow Push ups – On the wall, against the coffee table or couch or down on your hands and knees. Keep your hands wide and lower to ninety degrees at the elbow.

Commercial # 4. V- Sits – Sit on the edge of your chair/sofa, cross your arms over your chest, keep your back straight, engage your abs and lean back and hold for ten seconds and sit back up tall. Next time place hands at your temples and then complete the rest with the arms overhead.

My goal is to get you moving more than the time that you spend sitting. Of course, if you have any health conditions that would limit your ability to do the above exercises, it is best to listen to your body and do what feels right for you. Maybe that means just marching on the spot during the commercials. Either way, stand up and move.

Beth

# THE IMPORTANCE OF FITNESS TOOLS

January 25, 2019

Electronic fitness trackers. Fitbits. Apple watches. Old fashioned step counters. For some people, these devices play an important role in keeping them on point when it comes to exercise. I'm thrilled when people come up to me with smiles on their faces after class to tell me how many 'steps' they just completed! I was quite skeptical of these gadgets when they first came on the market but I learned a long time ago, that the real goal is to get people moving and whatever accomplishes this qualifies as an excellent fitness tool.

I see people fall off the fitness wagon regularly and my job is to motivate, encourage and to do all I can to ensure that people stay on track because quite honestly, our health is the most important thing we own. And it must be maintained by consistent effort or it slips away easily.

This is why I have invested in so many different pieces of equipment over the years for my private students to use when training. I am trying to keep people's interest. It is also why I keep studying. I hold a number of certifications so that I can help people achieve their goals in any way that they would like to move!

I wrote a fitness book to try to reach even more people and the latest tool that I have added to my business are workout videos. I have made three separate videos; one for beginner, intermediate and advanced students. The response has been wonderful but I have a few people saying, "I don't need a video because I come to class!" This is a fair point but we can't always make it to class and far too often when people miss one, they miss two and are at risk of stopping altogether.

I made the videos for this reason. When the weather is bad or you have an appointment and have to miss the class time, you can stream one of the three videos offered and still exercise. And you can take me on vacation when you leave for the sunny spots three months at a time. Your body will thank you and there is less chance that you will fall off of the fitness wagon!

There are die hard gym participants and also people who swear by exercising at home. It is often hard to convince one to try the other but I always say that variety is key. Put many tools in your fitness tool box and give yourself the best chance at success.

You can find all of my videos and books at betholdfield.ca.

Beth

# SLEEPING IS A FAT BURNING ACTIVITY

June 28, 2016

Yes, it is true. According to Dr. Natasha Turner, we burn fat while we sleep. During an interview on the Marilyn Dennis Show, Dr. Turner called sleeping "a great fat burning activity." This caught me by surprise but of course it makes sense because our body repairs itself while in sleep mode. While this does not mean that you can cancel your gym membership and spend all day napping in bed, it does mean that if you are having trouble losing weight, maybe you are not getting enough sleep.

Most clients I know who are struggling with weight loss, have terrible sleep patterns. They generally go to bed very late and wake up often, before falling out of bed, groggy, the next morning. Lack of sleep can lead to cravings, which can lead to poor eating, which can lead to poor sleeping. It really is a vicious cycle. Dr. Turner explains how hormones are negatively affected by poor sleep and how this translates into weight gain.

I am not a doctor, so I will refrain from giving you any advice on how to get more sleep. I will tell you that you need to address poor sleep habits if you are struggling with weight loss. It is not always about what you can accomplish at the gym when it comes to losing weight. Look at where your calories are coming from, how stressed you are feeling and how well you are sleeping at night. If there is a problem with any one of these three things, then you need to seek help if you really want to lose weight. Dietitians and your family doctor are your best resource when it comes to learning how you can improve your sleep quality and your life balance. I can help you burn those extra calories once you climb out of bed and get to my class.

Beth

# IT TAKES THREE CLASSES

April 26, 2016

It takes at least three classes to get used to any new type of exercise program, so I always ask that students give me at least three chances before deciding if the workout is the right fit for their needs. The truth is, though I love meeting new clients, I am usually a bit nervous when I greet a newcomer to the gym and as a result, I might not give my best performance on your first day. By day two you will feel more comfortable with the flow of the class, but you won't have found your comfort zone just yet. The third time that we see each other is what I refer to as the sweet spot because you will feel like you belong and by this time you will have met a few students and will be well on your way to sticking to your commitment to improve your health.

It takes courage to walk into a room full of people when everyone seems to know exactly what to do, where to stand and how to set up the equipment! I am so grateful that I have caring students who take it upon themselves to welcome strangers and lend them a hand getting organized.

It takes time to achieve our goals and while I say that it takes at least three classes to feel comfortable in a class, it then takes a few weeks to start to see results. Please do not expect instant transformations as those only happen on television. While every workout won't be perfect, know that showing up is the hardest part and doing something is far better than doing nothing. Bravo!Beth

# ARE YOU FOCUSED?

November 4, 2016

Yesterday in class, I noticed several people who appeared to be distracted by their thoughts. I can tell when your mind is elsewhere and I want you to know that when I remind you to focus on what you are doing, I am not doing it to be funny, I am doing it to keep you safe. While I have said that working out makes us feel better no matter what we may be going through, this is only true if you leave your troubles at the door when entering.

I know that many of you are dealing with chronic pain that can be quite distracting. I know that some of you have recently lost loved ones which is incredibly challenging, and I know that some of you have major life changing events coming up in the near future. My concern is to keep you safe while you are in class and if you are not actually thinking about what you are doing, while you are doing it, you are more prone to injuries.

During a Step or Dance class you could trip and hurt yourself or the students around you. In muscle conditioning, you need to be focused on your posture and the exercise that you are doing, so that you avoid moving in the wrong way. I often clap or snap to move you out of your reverie and draw your attention back to the task at hand. Sometimes, if I am really concerned, I will call out your name and make a joke. Just know that I am doing this to remind you that you are in class and you need to be fully present. The next time you find that you are thinking about something other than your workout, take a deep breath and turn your focus back to your body. For that one hour, give your mind a break from the worry and center yourself on getting stronger and more flexible, all of which will help you to handle the challenges of life much easier.

Beth

# IF YOU CAN'T MEDITATE, CONCENTRATE

September 8, 2016

I continue to hear clients say that they just can't get into the meditation aspect of yoga and I can understand this perspective. The first time I experienced meditation, I was on a yoga retreat and we began the day together with an hour of meditation. I thought I was going to burst. I had never meditated before and was unprepared for this experience.

This yoga studio was located in Ottawa which is one and half hours from my home. I had risen at dawn and had rushed to make it there on time. I was pumped and ready to get moving but we were asked to be still for what seemed like an eternity. My mind would not slow down.

The leader had told us to try to resist the desire to shift our position or scratch those itchy places on our nose etc. She told us to focus on our breath and if we still could not settle, she asked us to isolate one sound in the distance and focus on that instead. You know what happens when someone tells you that you can't move or scratch? I was suddenly itchy and felt the need to fidget non-stop. It felt terrible so I can understand it when people tell me that they will never be able to meditate. If you are one of those people, maybe you can think of this aspect of yoga as 'concentration' instead of 'meditation.'

In all fitness activities, you will benefit far more from the exercise at hand if you really concentrate on where you are, and what you are doing, in that very moment. If I teach you how to perform a squat, hopefully you're going to really concentrate on doing it well so you don't get injured.

If you are lying on your back, and I ask you to meditate, concentrate on your breathing. People generally only breathe into the top third of their lung capacity. Focus on breathing better. Equate it to any other exercise you would do at the gym. Your challenge is to do it to the best of your ability and eventually you will be able to concentrate for longer periods of time on other activities in life.

While holding the yoga poses, the idea is to not entertain every thought about your discomfort. Acknowledge that you feel your muscles but don't give into the idea of giving up because it is hard. Try not to scratch those itchy spots for the duration of the pose. Try not to think about anything other than your breath. This exercise is about controlling your thoughts so they do not control you.

Eventually our yoga practice helps us to handle events that come our way, over which we have no control. We learn to keep our thoughts in the here and now and focus on what needs to be done to survive whatever comes our way, including the next yoga class!

Beth

# NEW WORKOUT BLUES

February 2, 2016

It is a new month, which means new programs for all of my students. Today, I introduced the new routines to many of my classes (each routine being different, as I teach all different levels of fitness) and there was quite a bit of grumbling going around the room.

Yes, I know that it is hard to learn new exercises but the whole point is that you have mastered the January programs and now it is time to change things around. We want to switch up the way we work out to prevent overuse injuries and to avoid the dreaded plateau effect. When we always train in exactly the same way, our bodies adapt and then we stop seeing results.

I try to build on the skills that you have mastered over the month by increasing the difficulty slightly. Your body is then forced to 'work' again. You will burn more calories and increase strength and flexibility. We are working hard on our balance so there were many reasons for the grumbling today. Perhaps you discovered areas of your physical fitness that need improving. This can make us feel a bit down but remember that we felt this way one month ago. Many of us had a month off over the holidays, so that first week back was quite challenging. I have every confidence that you will love this new program as much as the last one.

Beth

# IF IT HURTS, YOU'RE DOING IT WRONG

September 18, 2019

There is a certain amount of discomfort that we must endure in order to get into shape but if you're experiencing intense pain during your workouts then we need to talk. You can't possibly focus on proper posture and technique when your brain is sending you pain messages and that worries me because this puts you at risk for injury in your back, knees and shoulders.

There is a certain amount of bravado that occurs in a group fitness class. No one wants to look like they need to stop even if they're hurting, but I encourage you to seek out ways to exercise pain free so that you can get the most out of your training session. For instance, one of my clients has been experiencing foot pain lately for various reasons. I suggested doing most of her workout from a seated position so that she could then be mindful of posture and focus on working her upper body muscles well, until her foot issues go away.

I don't want people to stop exercising altogether because it's too easy to fall out of a fitness routine and lose the benefits that we have gained. Instead, I encourage the use of props like thera-bands to lift your leg when you need to pull it behind you to do a quadriceps stretch if your shoulder or knee is bothering you; yoga blocks to lift your buttocks higher off of the ground so that you can take the pressure off your lower back when in a seated position on the floor, or the block can help you to reach the floor when you're doing a standing forward fold. You can place a cushion under your head to relieve neck pain during your mat work and you can do almost any upper body exercise effectively while seated in a chair if you have a knee, hip or leg injury.

We need to keep moving but we need to be smart about it. It's normal to feel that fitness is difficult but if the only thought you're having while exercising is how painful it is then speak to me to see if I can help to relieve your discomfort. Ultimately you should feel better after a workout, not worse. Let me know how I can help.

Beth

# WATCH THOSE KNEES

November 14, 2018

I tell my students to let me know if they feel any pain during our exercises and one of the most common types of discomfort that I hear about comes from the knees. As fitness professionals, we are not allowed to diagnose pain but we can make some suggestions on how to deal with it when it arises.

My first piece of advice is to seek the support of a physiotherapist so that they can tell you the probable cause and guide you on how to avoid making the situation worse. It actually surprises me how many people refuse to go and get their knees looked at by a physio. For some people, it's the cost that deters them, which is understandable to a certain extent, but I cannot stress enough how important it is to listen to your body as those pain signals are like the squeaks you hear in your car brakes before the pads are completely ineffective. Before real, long lasting damage is done, see the 'knee mechanic' and start following their advice and you might be able to avoid a far worse situation in the future.

What I hear most often is, "Oh I will be fine. It just occurs once in a while when I ..." and you can fill one of many statements to finish the sentence. "When I climb stairs, run, do aerobics, dance, squat or lunge." It is good to take note of when you feel the pain because that will give your physio clues as to what might be going wrong within the joint. For example, if you are used to always moving forward, aerobics might aggravate weaknesses in your knees because of the lateral (side to side) motion. Our joints become strong or weak based on the types of activities that we are doing on a regular basis. We need to strengthen the whole joint to work against these imbalances and that is what the physio does.

So when I hear people say they won't go to the doctor or physiotherapist that leaves me with just one suggestion which you hear me say all of the time. "If it hurts stop doing the movement and work in a pain free range of motion." Nine times out of ten, clients will continue to do the exercise which concerns me. While it is normal to have a tough time performing that last squat or lunge, you should not be feeling an intense sting of a suffering knee joint. Your body is telling you to stop and it is best to listen.

Another reason people refuse to seek medical treatment is the fear that they will be told that they must stop the activity that they love. I love to run but when I tried to take it back up this past summer, my ankles refused to participate properly and I ended up re-injuring my Achilles heel and had to give up both running and teaching Step. My physio had told me years ago that running was out of the question simply because of my situation but I chose to ignore her and now I have paid the price.

My last piece of advice is to watch your knee alignment in your group exercise classes because you might be rushing and improper positioning can cause undue pain. If you need any help with this ask your instructor to check your stance. That is something we can do to help but the rest is up to you! You must listen to your body.

Beth

# TELL ME WHAT YOU DON'T LIKE

March 6, 2017

When clients tell me what they don't like doing in fitness classes, I pay attention and then I do my best to incorporate some of those dislikes into our sessions together. I know that this sounds a bit bizarre but my goal is to help my students to improve.

Presumably, we all love to do the exercises that we're good at because we feel successful and strong. My job as your trainer, whether we are working together one-on-one or in a room with fifty other students, is to improve weaknesses. For instance, if you happen to mention to me that you hate balance challenges, then my guess is that this is because you feel you have a weakness in this area. I then know that we need to incorporate more balance training, so that you don't suffer a serious injury from a fall. While I cannot guarantee that exercises to improve your balance will prevent falls altogether, I can work on improving your core strength to lessen the impact, should you stumble.

I have clients who have told me that they absolutely hate push-ups. After a bit more discussion, I discover that the real reason is usually that they feel they cannot do them well. My goal at that point is to strengthen all of the muscles used for this exercise and then have them do one or two well and before we know it, they have improved and now feel better about push-ups. They may still 'hate' them but now it is for a different reason: repetitions!

A large percentage of my male students hate devoting time to stretching. This is usually because they feel unsuccessful. I do my best to work stretching into any fitness program for these clients. I spend at least ten minutes at the end of each group fitness class stretching to help everyone improve their flexibility and I always tell my clients with tight muscles to join a yoga class. Tight muscles lead to injuries later in life.

I have met clients who have tried my line dance classes and they have given up after only one experience. Now some students may simply hate the music or the fact that they have to follow a pattern, because they just want to bust into their own moves, but more often than not, it's because they are having trouble with their memory. I have watched clients in this situation improve their memory skills to such an extent that they now can correct me if I make a mistake!

Think about the components of fitness that you hate because they are highlighting a weakness that when improved will result in better health.

Beth

# IS YOUR CORE STRONG ENOUGH?

January 21, 2016

At this time of the year, all of my students, in all of my classes are working on developing their stability muscles. All of us need to be ready for slippery walking conditions. My hope is that by developing our core muscles and leg strength, we will be ready to catch ourselves when we slip on the ice and if we do fall, that we will be strong enough to get back up. I prepare my students all year to have a strong core but I incorporate even more exercises in the winter months to make sure that they are ready for that inevitable sidewalk slip!

One of the best ways to prepare our bodies for potential falls is to train on one leg, so we often have one knee lifted when we are standing and doing weight lifting. This activates all of the stabilizer muscles and gets them practiced at doing their job! We often use a disc that slides on the floor. One foot is placed upon the disc and we gently push the disc backwards which brings us into a lunge position. I then cue my students to use the front leg only to get themselves back up into an upright position.

"Pretend that you have slipped on ice and that the back foot is of no use to you. Use your front leg only to get yourself back upright." Of course there are plenty of other instructions to go along with this but for those you have to come to class! I do this to make sure that they are strong enough on one leg to get themselves up if one of their legs is hurt after a fall.

I have a very personal reason for doing all of this work toward fall prevention. When I was very young, a relative died at the bottom of her basement stairs. She lived alone in her later years and had taken a spill down the stairs. I have always wondered if perhaps she fell and simply could not get up to get help. She was found several days later.

Near the end of my dad's life, he was in a wheelchair. My mom had fallen coming out of the bathroom and she was unable to get up. My dad thought he could help if he got down on the floor and then they both laughed when they realized that they could not help each other to get back up. Somehow, they managed to call 911 and both of them had to be lifted up.

Of course, we do not have control over what the future holds for us. Part of my mission as a trainer is to help my students be stable enough to avoid falls, and strong enough to help themselves out of a serious situation, should they find themselves on the ground. I do this with all ages by the way, as we all need to be ready for the surprise of slipping. If we are not in shape, muscles can be injured, ligaments torn and bones can be broken. The truth is, the better shape that you are in before a fall, the shorter your recovery time will be.

One of my students, who is in his mid fifties, just told me yesterday of how he avoided a serious fall during the last snowstorm. We were doing some one legged exercise and he mimicked how practising that particular exercise in class had prepared him for the slip. His core and his leg muscles remembered the moves that we had practised in class, so his body was ready to kick into action and prevent a serious injury! I love hearing these stories! They keep me going.

Beth

# COMPARE YOURSELF

December 10, 2015

I invited one of my personal training clients into one of my fitness classes this week. She was going to be working out on her own anyway, so I thought she might benefit from seeing what we do as a group.

I sometimes forget how powerful this experience can be for people. She spoke to me after the class and mentioned that she found the class quite challenging and when I listed off the ages of some of the people in the class, she was shocked. The students were either one year older than her, or twelve years older and they are extremely fit. She now realizes that she has been staying in her comfort zone, to her own detriment. You see she was very averse to the attempts that I was making to increase the challenge of her workouts. She had a hard time doing many of the exercises that I do with this demographic regularly. This was a good wake up call.

Be honest with yourself. Have you settled into a routine that is keeping you from exploring new challenges? Has the workout regime become too easy? Have you slipped into a comfort zone and fooled yourself into thinking that you are in shape, when in reality you have stopped progressing and improving? While I tell my clients to always listen to their own bodies and not judge themselves based on the performance of others, I need to add that it is also good to measure our fitness level by attending some classes that we don't normally attend. This way we can see what others are doing and how we measure up compared to others our age. I have clients in their eighties who are fitter than some of my forty-year-old students. Do some exploring!

Beth

# MUSCLE SORENESS - ARE YOU PREPARED?

November 25, 2015

Delayed Onset Muscle Soreness or DOMS can be felt anywhere from one to three days after exercise. It catches us off guard in that way because we often cannot remember what we did specifically to cause the reaction. I do not often experience DOMS because I am careful not to push myself too hard, however on Monday evening during my Yoga Stretch class, I deviated from my 'lesson plan' and added a stretch that I had not done in over two years. I was feeling very good and I decided to challenge myself and the class.

Well, the soreness started last night and I only just put two and two together. Even though this is my career, I had forgotten that this is the body's normal reaction to being pushed a bit too far. Instead of linking it to one of my classes, I started to imagine that I was experiencing the symptoms of some life threatening disease. It is funny how our mind sometimes races to the worst case scenarios. I can see how worried my clients are when they tell me about their DOMS. They are very concerned that this discomfort will be with them forever and that they may have done some permanent damage.

I always tell my students to do what feels right for them. This may mean only returning to exercise once the discomfort disappears, which is usually after a few days. I encourage walking and low intensity activity, hot baths or sauna. A massage may also help. In a short time, you should be able to resume exercise.

What I have learned from this experience is that I have not personally taken myself out of my comfort zone in a long while.

I gear all of my workouts to my students and I need to get back to taking the time to work out on my own. I will repeat the stretch that has caused this muscle soreness but in a more controlled and gentle way. I simply had not done it in a long time and so my body is speaking to me this morning.

I hope this helps you to know the difference between soreness and injury. While it is normal to feel a bit stiff after a change in your workout, intense pain that keeps you awake at night is not. DOMS rarely causes sleep disruptions. When you are at rest, you should not feel the soreness. It can take up to seven days for all of the soreness to disappear, however I really believe that being moderately active will help you recover sooner.

I tease my students and tell them that if they are experiencing DOMS, to come to class and let me know. This is far better than 'staying home on the couch and crying into a bag of potato chips!' Which is what I would want to do too...but don't.

Beth

# OPTIONAL MUSCLES?

May 22, 2019

Most of us would agree that working out is the key to good health. Anyone who has stopped their fitness regime for a few weeks or months will be the first to remark how much better they feel once they return to the gym. My question to you today is, are you moving every muscle that you have in your body the way it was designed to move?

Whether you attend formal fitness classes or work out in the comfort of your own home, I want you to be your own advocate this week and analyze the classes that you are attending. Are you doing the same exercises each time you go to the gym? Are you always working to the front of your body but never to the back or to the side? If so you might be setting yourself up for injury even though you are being proactive and working out!

There are over 600 muscles in the human body and none of them are optional. In fact, most of the time it is the smaller, lesser worked muscles that get weak and break down, resulting in pain and occasional expensive physiotherapy. Think of your car and how optimally it performs when all of the components are running smoothly and conversely how just one tiny part can cause a breakdown resulting in lost hours at work and expensive repairs.

You want to move every muscle in your body regularly, the way it was designed to move. When we only train certain muscles by doing the popular exercises such as squats, push-ups and abdominal crunches we ignore the rest of the muscles around those joints and can end up with knee problems, shoulder issues and back pain. For example if we overtrain the rectus abdominus, the 'six pack' muscle, we can pull our pelvis out of alignment and remove the key curve in our lower back that helps to absorb shock during daily activities. We need to work the entire core which involves all of the abdominal muscles and back muscles, not just the ones that give you a washboard stomach!

I am glad that you are at the gym but I want you to be aware that variety is the real key to good health. If you feel like the classes you are attending are too repetitive in their programming, switch up your routine. Remember that it is not just about strength but flexibility as well. Muscles that are trained regularly also need to be equally flexible because they will pull the joint out of alignment which will throw the whole muscle chain out of balance.

This is one of the most common complaints I hear, "I don't understand it. I used to be able to do *xyz* and now I can't?"

Repetition will cause injury if there is not an equal amount of time spent on the opposing movement. If you are rarely doing any exercises for your back, it will give out eventually. If we stop moving in a certain way, eventually we will not be able to move that way anymore because of atrophied, tight, weak muscles. So my message today is to analyze your current regime and see if you are working out in a balanced fashion. And if you have concerns speak to your trainer. Reach out if you have questions. I am happy to help.

Bravo for getting to the gym and see you soon!

Beth

# TEN POUNDS MAKES ALL THE DIFFERENCE

April 17, 2019

Most of us have experienced that moment when you go to put on a pair of pants that used to fit perfectly but now is uncomfortably tight. Often this is the first time that we notice we have put on a few pounds. Sure we may see the weight gain when we are quickly glancing in the mirror but until it starts to affect how we dress or how we move, most of us go about our day pleasantly unaware of those extra ten pounds.

For me, as small as I am, I noticed when I had put on 17 pounds. I had changed my workout regime and taken out most of the cardio component but I kept eating as if I was being as active, and the result was clear. My clothes were not fitting and then I started to feel a difference in my ability to call my dance classes. I was out of breath and that forced me to take a good, honest look at my behavior.

I am happy to report that the changes I have made this winter to my training regime have helped me to lose nine lbs and I am hoping to lose three more! Tabata training has made the difference. This high intensity cardio workout is an excellent way to improve your cardiovascular conditioning and burn calories.

Because I am small to begin with, people wrongly assume that I have 'room' to expand but the truth is I run the same risk of developing joint problems and disease as everyone else. What is frustrating for me is if I try to commiserate with people larger than myself about weight gain, I get chastised for having the audacity to complain that I feel fat. I can only assume that people mean well when they say, "You don't need to lose weight! You should gain a few pounds."

The truth is we all need to watch our weight and be proactive about our health, no matter what size we are. So when you start to see changes in your ability to move in a pain-free manner or when your clothes become tighter, have an honest conversation with yourself and decide what you want to do about it. You can choose to make a difference in your health. I am not saying it will be easy, but the choice is yours!

Beth

# HOW'S YOUR EXERCISE BUZZ?

October 2, 2019

Fitness does feel good and it will give you a natural high if you do it often enough and under proper guidance. Participating in formal exercise in a gym with a certified group fitness instructor or personal trainer, who gets your heart pumping and muscles working will be energizing. Some people refer to this sensation as a workout 'buzz.'

If you can exercise two to three days a week, for a month, you will begin to experience the workout buzz and you will actually start to crave exercise as a way to relieve stress and improve your mood. The problem I face as a fitness instructor is getting people to commit to attending classes, without fail, for months at a time, so that they can feel this buzz and reap the benefits.

Today's blog is just a reminder that if you truly want to live your best life, you have to put your health first. If you are tired of feeling tired and want to rid yourself of pain and be able to participate fully in your favourite activities, you need to make yourself a priority. Yes, I realize that life gets in the way sometimes. I am just here to remind you that missing two or three classes in a row is a slippery slope and can lead to you giving up completely because you never really reach the moment where you feel the buzz.

Once you truly see how much better you feel and find the joy of fitness for yourself, you will be asking me to give you more and that's what I live for! Please just get moving. There are so many options today to help you to get fit. Pick one today and get started.

Beth

# THREE TIPS FOR EXERCISING IN THE HEAT

July 4, 2018

It's normal to sweat during a workout. That's how the body cools itself down. We are experiencing quite the heat wave where I live, with daytime temperatures averaging 35° Celsius and I have had a number of people ask me if it's safe to exercise in the heat. If you're healthy and regularly participate in fitness classes, I see no reason why you should stop moving as long as you take three things into account:

1.  You might be dehydrated before heading to the gym. Simply existing in high heat causes us to sweat and lose water. If you drink very little water as it is, chances are you will be running at a deficit before you even begin to exercise. If you are dehydrated your body will not be able to produce the sweat needed to cool your skin down. This can be serious and might lead to heat exhaustion. Make sure to bring water to your class and to take sips every 15 minutes or so. Make sure you have water after the workout as well to replace the water you lost during the session. Avoid caffeine and alcohol as they are dehydrating.

2.  Wear light clothing. Most of us have our favourite workout gear and many women in particular hide their curves under long pants and thick t-shirts. You need to shed the heat that we generate especially when the temperature outside is so high. Choose clothing that is light and breathes well.

3.  Slow down the pace. Now is not the time to take your first outdoor boot camp class. I say this because you want to be able to properly monitor your experience and if you are new to the class, you will be unfamiliar with what to

expect. Do your regular workout but realize that you are going to move slower because of the heat and be patient with yourself. Work out for a shorter amount of time and if you start to feel unwell, speak to the trainer or gym monitor.

As a trainer I plan to change my plans for this week. I don't want to push my students in this weather. If we usually do a high intensity workout, I will make alterations to keep everyone safe. Sometimes I take advantage of the warm weather and do flexibility training. Gentle Yoga and Restorative Essentrics® are perfect activities for these hot summer days!

Stay safe and keep moving. In Canada, we long for this weather mid-winter. Enjoy it!

Beth

# THE KEY IS CHANGE

April 14, 2016

I had a client come up to me on Monday morning and tell me that she had just read an article that said we should stop doing aerobics and sit-ups and only do High Intensity Interval Training (HIIT). My first piece of advice is to be careful of extremes in exercise. While I agree that HIIT is effective for many people, it is not necessarily safe for everyone. Instead of simply following a trend in the industry, vary your workout and give new crazes a try to see if they are right for you but don't immediately give up something simply based on an extreme viewpoint.

What I am more concerned about is people falling into the trap of training exactly the same way while expecting their weight and body composition to change. If you want to see an improvement in your health, you must regularly increase the intensity or switch up your program. Simply trying something new can bring about amazing results but this doesn't mean that the 'old' program was wrong, it simply means that you had hit a plateau.

Improvements happen quickly in clients who go from doing absolutely nothing, to working out at the gym every day. Those individuals see dramatic changes in their weight and the way that their clothes fit, if they are watching what they eat as well. The trouble begins when they settle into that class that they love and keep doing only that for the next fifteen years.

I encourage you to try all of the different types of classes that are offered at your local gym. Listen to how your body responds to the training and adjust accordingly but be careful of labelling an entire workout regime bad. There is almost always something good in all forms of fitness. The key is change. Switch up what you are doing and you will see results.

# THE CYCLE OF PAIN

September 5, 2018

If you are a fitness enthusiast, you know that when we are inactive for long periods of time, our body stiffens up and simply performing daily activities can bring on a certain amount of pain. Ironically, when we work out too hard at the gym we also experience a bit of muscle soreness that can be painful. If we don't exercise at all, we can experience injuries because of weak muscles and loose joints that can lead to serious pain. I often hear people say that they cannot take part in fitness "because it hurts their knees and/or back too much!"

The pain experience is different for everyone. Some people believe that 'the burn' they experience the day after a class means that they got a great workout, whereas another person might hate it and blame the teacher for their muscle soreness. While it is normal to experience Delayed Onset of Muscle Soreness (DOMS), 24 to 72 hours after a workout, this pain will be enough to turn some people completely off exercise.

This cycle of pain plays a big role in my life because I am always trying to find ways to make the class experience fun and yet challenging at the same time, knowing that if some people find it 'painful' they will not return. Conversely, if it appears to be too easy, others will opt out. My goal as a group fitness instructor is client retention. I want people to come back! This is why it is important that clients read the class descriptions so they get exactly what they are looking for in a workout.

I always tell my clients to inform me before the class if they are experiencing any pain so that I can offer alternative exercises based on their situation. This will help them to enjoy the class, however my advice is to consult a doctor or better yet, a physiotherapist, regarding any persistent pain. Chances are that exercise will be recommended and the cycle continues!

If you are one of my regular students you are probably feeling stiff and you know that when we get back to regular classes, we will experience some pain but the 'good' kind! The kind that says we are moving once again. It is usually completely gone by the following week when we start feeling years younger, which is our ultimate desire! The truth is if you stay consistent with a fitness routine you will start feeling better with each passing day and if you have never done formal exercise, you actually don't know how good you could feel, so get started today!

Looking forward to seeing you all soon!

Beth

# IT'S ALL ABOUT MAINTENANCE

September 15, 2016

At some point in our lives we begin to focus less on trying to look like the pictures in magazines and more on maintaining our health. A client came up to me this week and told me that she is at this stage in her life and I reassured her that she is in the right class!

A few years ago I stopped trying to be the strongest person in the room and decided to help my students be the best that they can be. My goal is to teach my students proper technique and keep them functionally fit. I choose exercises that strengthen or lengthen the muscles that my students use most often in their daily activities.

People show up in my classes for many different reasons. Many want to lose weight but most simply want to stop the clock. I can honestly say that those students who have been in my classes for almost twenty years, have not aged at all. They look as good, if not better than they did when we first met and this is because they make fitness a priority.

Regular maintenance is something that we are used to doing on our cars or around our home. Maintaining your physical health should be on your To Do list. A lifetime of neglect cannot be addressed in one or two workouts a month or a year. We have to make formal exercise a part of our day.

See you in class!

Beth

# TRAIN FOR WINTER SPORTS IN SUMMER

September 21, 2015

The weather is definitely changing. My oldest son, who loves the winter, showed up at our house yesterday wearing his tuque and he will wear it until next Spring. He has taken off the baseball cap and is now getting ready for Winter. I know that this seems a bit early but in reality, if you are a winter sports enthusiast, now is the time to start training for your favourite winter sport.

I know of a few men who gather once a week during the cold winter months to play an hour or two of hockey. There are also Old Timer leagues in some towns, for players who are over thirty years old. My concern with both of these groups is that very few of the players spend any real time at the gym training for their sport. They then jump onto the ice and push themselves too fast, too hard and some end up getting badly injured.

My advice for you today is to join your local gym and start using the treadmill or join an aerobics class to improve your cardio before you lace up your skates. Follow that up with some muscular conditioning and stretching. By the time the outdoor rink is ready, you will be in fine form and ready to be the best at your favourite game.

When you start training under safe conditions, you can then see how your body responds and address any issues that might arise. Don't assume that because you were the best player last year or the year before, that your body today will be ready to respond the same way. Regularly test your limits in a safe way. Get to know what a good workout feels like so that if you start having a health crisis of any kind, you will know your body well enough to seek attention and help quickly, instead of ignoring your symptoms for the sake of the game and your friends. Be safe.

# YOUR FAVOURITE WORKOUT MIGHT BE THE PROBLEM

February 9, 2016

If you are training exactly the same way, every day, you are going to get hurt.

Yesterday, I had a few clients come up to me complaining about shoulder pain and/or knee pain. Now this was in my group fitness class and I only see these clients once per week. I of course cautioned them to always listen to their body and if something hurts, to not push through any pain but to stop immediately and if the pain persists, to see a doctor.

I know that many of you go to a number of classes per week, which is fine, but if you are doing squats in every single class, you are at risk for injuring your knee. If you are doing military press every single day, you will injure your shoulder. You must leave a day in between training muscle groups, to allow for rest and recovery and growth. If you are not affording your body the chance to heal, then you are overusing the joint and may injure yourself. If you attend my classes every day, than I make sure that what we do on Monday is different from what we do on Tuesday etc.

There are many teachers and many types of classes in our facility so it would be impossible for all teachers to know what the others are doing and to co-ordinate the muscle groups being worked. Therefore be proactive in your approach and if you see that the teacher has a muscle group planned that you did yesterday, ask for an alternative or use lighter weights or no weights or do another exercise altogether. I hate hearing that people are developing injuries when they are gym regulars but it can be avoided with some proper planning. Be mindful of what you are doing in each class and try to build in variety as you can. Reach out if you need some suggestions.

# PART THREE

# WISE WORDS FOR THE 50+ CROWD

**F**our years into my career I was offered the opportunity to teach seniors during the day instead of leading fitness classes in the evening. I jumped at this chance because at the time I had three young children at home and my husband and I were tag teaming at a grueling pace. He would rush home from work, (fifty plus kilometers) where I would pass the baton of childcare over to him and rush back out to the gym in Pointe Claire (fifty-two kilometers door to door) where I would work until 9 pm at night.

My boss at the time and mentor Shawna Lambert needed a replacement because one of the daytime teachers was retiring. I suggested that it was going to be hard to leave my nighttime students behind to which she suggested that we start an Early Bird class at 6:45am so they could keep training with me but in the morning before work. I am happy to say that more than a few students were thrilled to change their workout regime and the rest is history. I worked at that same location exclusively for twenty years. I absolutely loved working with the 50+ crowd during the day. They were happy to see me and eager to learn about my family and life and their devotion and energy has carried me through to this day.

Switching from nighttime to daytime fitness classes was the best decision I have ever made. I am passionate about this dedicated group of individuals and the following section highlights the blog posts that I wrote with this demographic in mind, though I encourage everyone to read on.

# FIGHT THE EFFECT OF GRAVITY

February 19, 2020

One of my favourite positions in Essentrics®, which is a dynamic stretching and strengthening workout that targets all 650 muscles and 360 joints in one class, is called Neutral Elongation. It is excellent at fighting the effect that gravity takes on our spine over time.

The truth is because of our largely sedentary life (I just stood up to finish writing this post) our posture tends to go from straight to forward leaning. Gravitational forces are constantly pulling us downward, so our poor postural habits, coupled with weak, atrophied core and back muscles, can contribute to neck and back pain.

I want you to give this posture correcting exercise a try. Stand with your feet hip width apart. Lift your shoulders up toward your ears and then roll them backward and down, feeling your shoulder blades slide down your rib cage. Imagine that you are putting your shoulder blades into your back pockets. Then remind yourself that your chin should be back so that your neck is lined up over your spine. Already this pose will feel like work because most of us do not stand or sit with proper posture and as a result our back muscles have become very weak.

As you inhale, I want you to let your arms float up in front of you, bending them at the elbow, and then raise them overhead. Exhale and slowly straighten your arms, while gently depressing your shoulders at the same time. Your arms should be lined up with your ears but that can be very hard for some people, so just lift your arms upward in a pain-free range of motion.

Now slowly reach for the ceiling, one arm at a time, keeping your eyes forward. I want you to reach up for a count of three, until you feel you can go no higher but then relax and wait a

114

second and see if you can get just a bit higher. Repeat with the opposite arm. Now repeat with both arms at the same time, inhaling and then as you exhale, lower your arms out to the side, gently pushing your palms away as if you are pushing walls away. Try to open your chest as you lower the arms, bringing the elbows slightly behind the shoulders. Complete this exercise three times in a row if time permits.

Do this exercise every day if you can and in time, you should see a change in your posture which should alleviate back and neck pain.

Beth

# RETIREMENT IS NOT THE TIME TO SLOW DOWN!

November 6, 2019

Many of my clients began training with me several times a week when they were working full time and because I have been around for so long, I have watched them transition into retirement. As a result, I have had a front row seat to seeing how differently people choose to retire. Most people downsize their living quarters and start travelling regularly to see family and friends. Many people take up new hobbies and sports and quite a few join the gym for the first time in their lives, to take better care of themselves.

Younger people often dream about retirement in a positive light. Better sleep. More time for sitting and reading and self care. While all of that is important I would argue that slowing down is the last thing that we want to do, especially after the age of 65.

Our bodies are designed to move and when we stop articulating each joint and muscle in the way in which it was designed to move, the body interprets this as us saying that we no longer need those muscles. If we stop performing certain physical movements, such as getting down on the floor or touching our toes, we will lose this ability because of muscular weakness and tightness and these imbalances will lead to a misaligned spine and eventual pain in our knees, hips and back. As Miranda Esmonde-White explains in her latest book, *Fast Track To Aging Backwards - 6 Ways and 30 Days to Look and Feel Younger,* "over time the body will stop making those movements available to us" (Esmonde-White, 2019, p. 15). A sedentary lifestyle is the quickest track to premature aging.

I now tell my students that we need to move every joint and every muscle daily, to keep those cells alive, refreshed and young. If we consider how bad it is to let a car sit for extended periods of time, without letting the engine run or the wheels turn, the same can be said of our body. In order to stay vital and be able to live our lives to the fullest, we need to become more active when we retire.

The good news is that once people stop working, they have more time to dedicate to physical fitness. Our goal should be to move more than we sit each day. I recommend a balanced program that includes weight bearing exercises and stretching.

Contact me if you would like a personalized program.

Beth

# INTERNATIONAL DAY OF OLDER PERSONS

October 2, 2017

Yesterday was the International Day of Older Persons. I had no idea that there was an annual day devoted to celebrating seniors but it happens every October 1st. It was created by the United Nations General Assembly and the first one was celebrated in 1991. This year the theme for the International Day of Older Persons was "Stepping into the Future: Tapping the Talents, Contributions and Participation of older persons in Society."

I do not see age when I look out upon the students in my classes. Instead I see many retired professionals from all different backgrounds, who finally have the time to dedicate to their own health. Once more these individuals are incredibly busy volunteering in their communities and helping their families.

The talent among my students is striking. I have several nurses in my midst, and former teachers, pilots, war veterans, doctors, nurses, lawyers, engineers, and accountants. A number of the former teachers get called back regularly to substitute teach and one former editor just can't seem to fully retire as new projects keep popping up into her life.

I am in awe of the energy that my students bring to class each day. Some are facing health struggles and/or suffering the loss of loved ones but I want all of my students to know that I recognize the unique contribution that you bring to society. I love hearing your wisdom. I get all kinds of wonderful advice and though I am often in a hurry, I hope that you know how much I appreciate the time that you take to speak to me and share your thoughts.

You are all so busy, sometimes I worry about retirement! It can be hard to nail many of you down as you fly between activities. Seniors are among the busiest people I know and they have the most to contribute to our society. I hope that my classes will keep you in shape so that you can continue to play an active part in your social circles.

Next year let's celebrate International Day of Older Persons together!

Beth

# TOO OLD TO LEARN?

June 5, 2019

Learning keeps us young. I see evidence of this every single day at the gym. I am glad that people are getting to my classes because this is one of the best ways to slow the aging process but today's blog is a heads-up for my students. Even though you are devoted and attending regularly, I have noticed that the students who take the time to learn a new skill such as piano, knitting or choir seem be slowing the aging process even more!

What does this mean? How can I see it?

Don't forget that I have known many of my students for more than ten years and as such I have had a front row seat to watch them climb the birthday calendar. I can see that the clients of mine who are regularly engaged in learning a new sport, activity or hobby are better able to process information during a fitness class quickly and as such they are less likely to stumble or be thrown off balance! These students have a natural spark in their eyes and a bounce in their step. They move faster and this is despite the common injuries that tend to plague us all as we age, such as sore knees and stiff hips. Their attitude is positive and they are excited and ready to try new moves in class. To be clear, I am not criticizing the students who prefer to keep their lives low key, I just want to tell you that you can do even more to stay young in both the mind and the body!

I had the pleasure last week of watching my sister and her husband, who are in their late sixties, perform at a casual choir event in Ottawa. I was completely impressed by how motivated they were to be up there, front and center, singing their hearts out. It was an evening event, almost two hours from their home but this did not deter them in any way! Singing is great exercise for the lungs and they were grooving as well.

My line dancers challenge their minds by mastering compli-cated steps that force them to move fast on their feet. I can see how much this is helping them in life in general.

This summer, when our gym cuts the number of classes in half, why not fill those missing hours with a course that will teach you a new skill? Or a course that will add to your knowl-edge about your favourite subject. The idea is to challenge your mind, not just your body. We need to do both to stay young.

Beth

# THE BATTLE AGAINST DECOMPOSITION

September 28, 2016

Often we feel great until we reach too high, move a bit too fast or twist a bit too far. The hard truth is that we're all breaking down slowly and if we're not working hard at maintaining our health through regular formal fitness, then we're putting ourselves at risk of injury. I meet plenty of people who feel that they don't need to go to the gym because they feel stellar on the inside and look like they did when they were younger but looks can be deceiving.

Muscles shrink and become weak and tight if they are not used the way that they were designed to move. It's not enough to simply be active. Yes, you can play golf or swim or walk but the muscles that are **not** used during those activities are losing their ability to perform optimally. Your body is a chain and you need every link to keep working properly if you want to remain healthy.

Please don't be under the illusion that you can still run as fast as you once did or that you can lift as much weight, if you have not been exercising the whole body properly. Just because you were an athlete in high school, does not mean you are ready to jump hurdles or play rugby. The muscles needed to help us live active, functional lives, have to be moved properly, regularly. Aim to train all of the muscles in a balanced way through formal exercise with a certified trainer.

My client's range in age from mid fifty to early eighties and it is because of their dedication to formal fitness that they continue to enjoy healthy living. Contact me if you need some help.

Beth

# AGEISM DRIVES ME CRAZY!

January 7, 2016

In my work, I deal with a lot of ageism. People make judgements based on someone's age, rather than on ability. Perhaps because I grew up with older parents, I was socialized to be welcoming to everyone no matter their age and so it shocks me when I encounter disdain for older adults.

Some trainers don't want to be seen working with aged clients for fear that they will be thought of as 'too easy' a trainer. I actually giggle when I come across this attitude because honestly working with this demographic has given me such joy that I feel I have a little secret that I am happy to keep to myself. Yes, they are older but they are also kinder, accepting, loyal, invested and engaged in all aspects of the class. They want to be there and they are eager to be challenged. I work with some clients in their 40's who are not as fit as my 70-year-old students!

What shocks me the most, are those clients who refuse to attend some of my classes, because they are filled with students who have white hair. They have told me that they simply do not want to be seen with old people when in reality every person, no matter their age, can work to their level within any of my classes. This is how you should approach any fitness class. Yes, look around to see how everyone is doing but at the end of the day, it is you who must put in the work to your own level. It shouldn't matter whether the person beside you is 70 or 30. The truth is my students look as young as they did when I first met them. I am so motivated by the fact that regular fitness has seemingly stopped the clock when it comes to aging.

Aging is nothing to fear. It is something to celebrate and embrace.

Beth

# EMBRACE THE NEW NORMAL

November 6, 2017

I have had the privilege of watching my students handle the process of aging over many years and the number one mistake that I see is people avoiding the subtle and not subtle ways in which their body is communicating that real change is needed. Just because you have always done something does not mean that you should keep doing it, especially if your body is hurting. I am referring specifically to knee and shoulder injuries.

I see over one hundred students a day and you would not believe the number of people who are grappling with physical changes but not working toward finding a solution to the problem. How many of you reading this right now have a nagging pain in one of your joints that you are not addressing because it may mean you have to change your activities?

This is what I hear several times per week, "Oh it will go away if I just rest it a bit! I don't need to see a doctor or stop attending this class."

Keep in mind that insisting on doing the same activities simply because it is what you have always done, limits your potential to grow and find joy in living. Should you find that your knee or hip or shoulder can no longer golf, curl, jog, or perform the way it used to, you owe it to yourself to seek healing help, but then also to explore other options for keeping fit. For example, water aerobics, yoga and Essentrics® are typically easier on the joints and provide a great workout as well. Higher impact classes may be fun but they can be damaging over time so please embrace the way that your body is changing and make adaptions to stay safe and healthy!

Beth

# ARE YOU PREPARED?

May 13, 2015

Whether we are playing sports with friends or trying to keep up with grandchildren at the family BBQ, my mission is to make sure that my students are prepared for when things go wrong. While I can't prevent accidents from happening, my goal is to make sure that you are in such good shape when they do happen, that the impact on your life is minor, instead of major.

How many times have you lifted something beyond your abilities because you did not want to wait until someone was able to assist you? Or when was the last time you played frisbee or badminton? A simple game can take a toll on our muscles. All is fine and dandy until someone slips a disc in the lower back! For this reason, I do my best to improve your core strength through abdominal training and back exercises.

In class we focus on our balance, by lifting one leg while we are performing certain exercises. I build this challenge in regularly because I want the muscles that help you to restore your balance toned and ready to be called into action quickly. Icey sidewalks can catch us off guard but some health conditions can result in loss of vision which can be very destabilizing. A year or two before my Mom died, she lost her vision in one eye. Suddenly life became very difficult. We never know when we may need to have an operation on our eye and having good balance ahead of this, will certainly help to prevent falls.

I am always telling my students that we need to be able to lift ourselves off of the ground. Push-ups are so important. My Aunt died alone at the bottom of her basement stairs. She may have died suddenly from the fall or she may have suffered for days simply because she could not lift herself up. As a result of this tragedy, I incorporate triceps push ups into our classes. Try this: lie on your stomach with your hands right beside your chest, keep your elbows close by your side, and lift your chest and belly off of the ground, coming onto your knees. Being able to do this is beneficial and being able to do it more than once is good, as it often takes us several attempts to get up after a fall.

We should be able to defend ourselves. When I was young, my parents' minister and his wife died tragically after they were brutally attacked in their home. I will spare you the terrible details but this couple were elderly and my parents felt very vulnerable after this event. While I do not encourage violence, I have my students practice punching and kicking in our aerobics routines. Practice makes perfect and if you are used to doing something, your body will respond instinctively when needed. One of my students said she used to dream of punching and kicking and unfortunately her husband would get a rude awakening as the occasional leg or fist would fly across the bed. I guess she was practicing!

Please share your 'near disaster' stories with me as they help me to build solutions into my fitness programs. Last year one student, at the age of 75, had to use the fire escape to get out of her building. She was so proud to tell me that she was able to climb down! I get countless reports of doctors being amazed at the leg strength of my students not to mention their fabulous flexibility.

There is method behind my madness when it comes to program design and I really feel that it is important that you understand my reasoning. Always ask your trainer why they want you to do an exercise. Make sure that they know why it will help you to make your life better. If they have no answer, be wary of the intent. Make sure that the trainer has your best interests at heart!

Beth

# STRONGER THAN BEFORE AT EIGHT-FOUR!

January 25, 2017

"I'm 84 years old and stronger than I was before!" – Brigitta.

I met Brigitta in 2013 and when she introduced herself to me she took my breath away. She doesn't know this but she looks a little bit like my mother, who passed away in 2007. Brigitta is a very kind, soft spoken lady who rarely misses class and always wears a smile.

Yesterday, in the Ice Storm, Brigitta made it to my Chair Muscle Conditioning class along with eleven other students. I did not expect anyone to show up, as the news media was telling everyone to stay home, and I don't fault anyone for choosing to remain indoors. The sidewalks were skating rinks.

Brigitta walks to my class as she has no car, so I asked her if she had taken a lift this time.

"Oh no, I have a walking stick!" This warmed my heart and left me giving thanks that she had arrived safely. Brigitta told me that she believes the classes have developed her core to the point where she feels she is more stable, and better able to handle days like yesterday. In her own words, "Thank you for the health and fitness you have given me with your excellent and well thought-out exercises. I think I walk and sit differently now. You made me aware of my body."

This body awareness has allowed Brigitta to abandon a back belt that she bought years ago to help her with gardening. She told me yesterday that she has not needed that belt for a long time. She believes that the exercises that we do have taken away the need for any such aid.

Brigitta is strong, flexible and from what I can see, pain free. Though I must add that most of my students are pretty good at not complaining. They are thankful and usually smiling, no matter what life throws their way...even ice storms!

It is never too late to start training. I hope you will be motivated by Brigitta's story and join us.

Beth

# WHETHER YOU ARE 50 OR 70, IT IS NEVER TOO LATE TO START

June 10, 2015

If you are planning on living out the rest of your life in good health, I highly recommend this book, "What Makes Olga Run?" by Bruce Grierson. This is the story of Canadian Track and Field legend, Olga Kotelko, who took up the sport at age 77.

As I work primarily with people over the age of 50, I am deeply interested in hearing how the Boomers are redefining what it means to be a 'senior citizen.' My students are so fit that I constantly brag about their abilities to younger individuals. They are too shy to let me name them but Lady X, who is over 80, can hold a plank on her elbows and toes, using a stability ball, for one minute, in perfect form I might add.

I have clients well into their 70's who can Step at 128 bpm for 30 minutes while performing complicated choreography. All of them have excellent balance and abdominal strength that far surpasses a lot of 30 year old's.

I have line dancers who can remember 64 counts of fast moving choreography, with tags and re-starts and spins! They often remind me when I have missed a move! Not to mention their flexibility! It is amazing.

Sadly though, this is not the norm. Most people give up on fitness altogether once they hit a certain age and that's when the quick decline happens in all aspects of health. If you are younger than 95 and feeling like you have missed your chance to be active, Olga's story will be uplifting.

Olga's achievements are unbelievable. Bruce gives us a candid look at Olga's life in an attempt to try to figure out what exactly made her so different from the rest of us. She held over 25 World Records in her age category and won over 700 gold medals, which according to Bruce she liked to give away to special individuals as she had "so many of them!"

Bruce lets you in on what Olga ate, how she trained and what her routines were. It's fascinating and some of the information may encourage you to "get off your butt," as Olga would say. I do not want to give away all of her secrets, I want you to read about her life yourself. I will tell you that Olga's main piece of advice is to keep moving.

My advice today, is to set physical goals for yourself. Goals that will keep you motivated to get off of the couch and move. How many times can you walk/run around the block? How long can you hold plank? How can you improve this? Set some personal goals this summer and have fun achieving them.

Olga insists that having goals gives us a reason to get outside and be with people. She lived until 95 in excellent physical health, beating records right up until the end. Olga was never a burden to anyone and is a wonderful reminder that age is just a number.

It is never too late to take up a new sport or activity. We are meant to inspire each other while we are here on this earth. Set one simple goal today and get moving.

Beth

# SENIORS WITH NOTHING TO DO?

April 17, 2017

I hear this comment quite a bit from younger people who try to describe retired individuals, "They have nothing to do and therefore all of the time in the world to do it!" Usually these words are being spoken by someone in their thirties or forties who has so much to do they can't see straight, however in my experience, seniors are some of the busiest folks I know!

I am fifty years old and work with retired individuals and I consider their time just as important as my own. It is true that retired seniors have lots of time to design their day but this does not mean that their time is any less valuable than the time of a working person. We are all working toward goals we hope to achieve. We are either working several jobs to buy the lifestyle that we desire, or we are now living the dream after years of hard work.

The seniors that I teach are quite busy volunteering in their community. They are taking classes and learning new skills, or they are involved with physical activities to keep themselves fit so that they can remain independent and healthy. Most of them take care of their grandchildren so that their kids can continue to work and save money.

Seniors are an integral part of society and their time is very valuable. While they may move slower simply because they are older, they are usually on their way to do important things. One of my students drives an hour out of her way to work at a rescue shelter for dogs. Many others work at the hospital in one capacity or another trying to ease the lives of patients.

Think twice before judging the person in front of you and have respect for their time.

Beth

# WHAT ABOUT YOUR BONES?

February 12, 2016

On Wednesday, I attended a moderated discussion at McGill with Dr. Lora Giangregorio, an associate professor in the department of Kinesiology, at the University of Waterloo. She was being honoured for her research into the use of exercise, in the management of osteoporosis.

"Bone disease affects more Canadians than heart attack, stroke and breast cancer combined." The problem is that we often do not know that we have an issue with our bones, until we fall and break something. Just because you do not fit the standard 'old decrepit person' profile, does not mean you get a free pass and can ignore your bones. You may have brittle bones because of diet, heredity or disease or menopause and not even know it.

I have been in the fitness industry, working out regularly for over 25 years so I was shocked to discover that I had osteopenia at the age of 48. I only found out because my doctor ordered a bone mineral density test, as a result of my gluten intolerance. My father who died in his 80's had osteoporosis but did not know it. We found out because of the autopsy.

The biggest lesson that I learned from Dr. Giangregorio, is that fitness professionals who deal with older adults (50 years old +), need to design group fitness programs that do not put their clients at risk. Dr. Giangregorio suggests weight training exercise two times per week, and she suggests implementing balance training for fall prevention. I am happy to say that I feel very confident about my programming after having attended this discussion. I want you to know that you are in good hands when you are attending my classes.

Beth

# DO YOU KNOW YOUR BASELINE?

May 24, 2017

One of my friends, Susan, just lost her 67-year-old brother. He died suddenly after not feeling well for a couple of weeks. I want to share her comment on the situation with all of you because I find it to be insightful. "Exercise is stressful and maybe if he had been attending a class regularly, he would have noticed something was wrong earlier."

Susan sees exercise as positive stress in the sense that it forces us to see potential problems before they develop. I believe that she is right. My students are very fit and they know when something is wrong because they have a baseline by which they can judge their health. For example, they know what it feels like to push themselves in an aerobic or muscle conditioning class and if they feel that suddenly they are unable to perform normally, it is worth checking in with the doctor. A gentleman that I was training in my home studio years ago knew there was something wrong when he could not catch his breath during our normal exercise class. He sought medical attention and was able to catch a serious situation before it grew worse.

Working out regularly not only keeps us in good shape but we become more aware of the quality of our health in the process. We learn to tell the difference between 'normal' discomfort and the feeling that something is very wrong with our health. While it might be a stretch to suggest that her brother could have been saved had he been exercising, I can see understand Susan's thought process. Once we know how good we can feel, we are quickly alerted to potential problems when we experience unusual sensations. Exercising regularly, helps us to understand ourselves and our body better which can help us to seek medical attention when something feels 'off.'

Another great reason to start training today. Let me know if I can help.

Beth

# SENIORS AND YOGA

May 4, 2016

Last Friday, I completed the Senior Yogafit training in Montreal. The course taught us how to bring yoga to people who would otherwise avoid it because most yoga classes take place on the mat, in bare feet. There is a huge percentage of the population who avoid getting down on the floor for fear that they will not be able to get up! There are also those who have pain in their feet and must use orthotics at all times to be balanced. It was refreshing to learn how to use various props in order to help these clients benefit from yoga postures.

In my Chair Yoga class we use a chair for the most of the course. One of my students was overjoyed to experienced yoga postures that did not put so much pressure on her knees and legs. She said that she was practically in tears when we were doing the Warrior poses seated! She was able to concentrate on expanding and stretching her upper body, instead of focusing on the pain in her legs.

This is the best part of YogaFit. As teachers we are taught to *make the pose fit the body, not the body fit the pose.* We do not push our clients into complicated postures if they are not flexible or fit enough and we do not make them feel badly if they cannot achieve the 'perfect' downward facing dog. Instead we encourage the use of blocks, chairs, blankets, bolsters and straps to bring the joy of yoga to everybody.

I see clients daily who are in chronic pain from having lived a full and exciting life. Most people have one spot or another on their body that gives them some sort of trouble. My goal is to relieve the stress that comes from dealing with pain, by teaching a class that is centered on making the student feel capable and successful. Using props and chairs enables everyone to feel that they can achieve yoga poses.

If there comes a time when you yourself suffer an injury or develop a condition that limits your mobility, do not be afraid to use props or the chair for your yoga practice. You will love it, I promise. You will reap all of the benefits of yoga without the pain!

Beth

# PROACTIVE FITNESS IS THE KEY!

April 3, 2017

My job as a fitness professional is to get people to exercise. Unfortunately, most of my friends, who range in age from 30 to 55, are too busy to get to the gym, so I spend quite a bit of time talking about the need to be proactive when it comes to our health. This makes me unpopular in some circles.

A few weeks ago, a client mentioned to me that they find my blog depressing because they are not old (59) and do not want to be thinking about avoiding things like dementia and falls at this point in their life. I could pull out statistics and give reasons for my approach from a scientific perspective, however to be honest most people tune this information out so I try to speak about what I see happening in the majority of my classes and with my friends.

How do I convince people that they need to make time for their health? Most people do not want to hear about the potential pitfalls of carrying too much weight. Most people do not want to hear that they are losing muscle mass and flexibility that will be hard to regain the longer they avoid formal exercise.

I am alarmed by the number of people experiencing chronic back, wrist and knee pain. I know so many people of all ages who fear that if they get down on the ground, they may not be able to get back up. I have young friends who cannot touch their toes, have no core strength and weak cardiovascular endurance.

I know that when an accident occurs, that these people will have a harder time recovering. The last thing I want is for my friends and family to suffer needlessly and this is why I hope that people decide to get to the gym before their doctor tells them that they need to lose twenty pounds for the sake of their knees, hips, backs and hearts.

What I know for sure, is that I want my students, family and friends to be able to move pain free, through a full range of motion. I want them to be able to get down on the floor and up again easily. I hope that they will be able to dance, play golf, curl and ski for as long as possible.

On a happy note. One of my most dedicated students just had knee surgery and she wrote to tell me how impressed the doctors were with her physical condition.

*"I am back home from the knee surgery, safe and sound. I have to thank you for the good shape my body is in. I surprised all in the hospital with my ability to lift and lower myself on one leg, getting up and sitting with ease, walking safely, not to mention the good bridge so they could stick the bed pan under me...I must say, that I think I am lucky with a high pain threshold. In the recovery room, the nurse was waiting for the pain to strike before sending me to the floor and luckily it never came... I am happy it all went better than expected. Now I have to work at bending the joint. The physiotherapist from CLSC is coming today. I feel strong, with all the narcotics gone, I have more pain but I hope to be able to do what I need to do.So again Beth, thank you for keeping us in shape!"*

Beth

# HELP A SENIOR

June 7, 2016

I teach a chair muscle conditioning class in which we often sit to lift our weights but we also use the chair for balance during the standing exercises. Despite the use of the chair, my students work very hard and they are fit! A funny thing happened last week that is still making me laugh and smile.

The building that I work in has an extensive children's program and there was an event for parents and their kids taking place beside my fitness room. I had left the room for a minute while the students were setting up their chairs and when I returned to sit down and get started, I noticed that there were several chairs set up but not in use in the middle of the room.

Whenever I notice an empty chair it concerns me, as it means that someone may have left in distress but the fact that there were ten empty chairs was bizarre. I asked everyone what was going on. The students started to laugh and explain that a young man, who was waiting in the hallway for the other program, came into our class and began setting up chairs at random. He had been watching my students take chairs off of the dolly and of course he saw that there was a need and he jumped in for the rescue. It was clear that he was trying to help and he had no idea that this was a fitness class.

We took a few minutes to giggle and then praise the young man for jumping to the aid of seniors but I had to ask my very fit crowd how often this happens to them in their daily lives? How often does someone younger offer to help them lift or carry something? Does this bother them?

What came out of the conversation was the message that they are not insulted when anyone offers assistance. Some seniors mentioned that it does not happen often enough, so when it does they are very grateful and they make certain to thank the person properly. It doesn't really matter if someone is helping you because they think you are 'too old' or 'too young' to handle something. What matters most is that people are offering to help one another.

This was a refreshing moment last week. Too often we are rushing and walking right by people in need. Taking a moment to smile and offer a hand to another human being makes everyone feel wonderful.

We need to do more of this!

Beth

# "WATER THE FLOWERS"

November 10, 2015

A close friend has said this to me many times as of late, "Water the flowers and forget about the weeds." In life we have to focus on the good things if we want to get more of them into our lives. I meet clients every day who spend a lot of time listing their various ailments to me. I am of course interested because I have to know that they have been cleared to exercise but sometimes I find that people are so consumed with what they perceive as their 'problems,' that they cannot see the good aspects of their situation. I often remind my students that we are so lucky to have the luxury of sweating together! We are not stuck in a hospital bed.

Last week during the stretching component of one of my classes, I heard a yelp for joy. I turned to find one of my students mastering that particular pose and she had a beautiful smile on her face. This great moment was a reminder to focus on the progress that we are making by regularly working out. I have some clients who give up on their goals because they expected success in three or four classes. They expected that if they stopped eating junk and showed up to work out every day for a week, they would lose twenty pounds and be instantly happy!

I am here to tell you that the progress will be slow at times but one day you will be able to touch your toes or you will find yourself pulling up those pants that used to be too tight. Focus on the little ways in which you are feeling stronger, healthier and happier. Just for a moment consider all that is right in your life and water those flowers!

Beth

# ARE YOU OLD?

July 16, 2015

In emails from two of my students yesterday, each of them referred to themselves as part of the 'oldies' club. One of the students is 63 and the other I am guessing is a bit older than that but to be honest, all of my students are in such good shape that I often cannot tell how old they are.

I remember last Spring one woman said her age out loud (80) during a conversation in a class that had 45 people in it and the collective gasp was audible, as everyone thought she was much younger. Then everyone broke into applause! I love these moments.

When I first started working with older adults I received the best piece of advice from Madeline Ramsay, a fellow instructor at my place of work, who was retiring. I was taking over her classes and she said to me, while wagging a finger in my face, "Don't you ever treat them like old people."

Many things can make us feel old and because I am in the fitness world, I know that one of these things can be trying a new class. Learning new moves with a different teacher can be challenging and frustrating. I do my best to make sure that everyone in the class can follow each move, as this builds confidence and ultimately the students will get better and stronger which makes us feel younger and more resilient.

One thing that I am extremely proud of is my ability to work with the 50 + crowd. Not many people know that I am trained to be an Older Adult Specialist along with all of my other certifications. Instead of simply arriving in a class to '"torture' my students so that they remember my name tomorrow morning, I arrive ready to take them along on a journey and this journey is totally geared toward their success

I received the best compliments after teaching my two yoga classes back to back last Friday. In the first hour a woman in her mid to late fifties, told me how much she enjoys my class because I really explain how to do the poses. Then in the second hour a much younger lady came up to me and said how grateful she is that I give students enough time in the poses, to actually get something out of them! She said that my class was the best yoga class she had taken. This made my day!

To me, it is not only about age but about learning. If students are not able to follow my cues, then I must adapt my teaching to suit their needs. If you leave my class feeling 'too old' to participate, then I have not done my job correctly. I do not consider any of my students to be old. I see no age. I only see bodies full of potential.

Thanks for sharing your experiences with me.

Beth

# REDEFINE YOUR AGE

April 4, 2016

If you are someone who is uncomfortable exercising beside a sixty year-old because you feel that you are too young to be in the same class, you had better get used to it because as Jo Ann Jenkins says in her book, *Disrupt Aging*, "10,000 people are turning sixty every day and this will happen for the next fourteen years."

When people make judgements about others based solely on their physical age, I cringe. It works both ways of course. It happens to young people fresh out of school who are looking for an employer to give them a chance, and it happens to older people who are considered to be past their prime. I have had young people (twenty-year old's) leave my classes because they do not want to be seen with sixty-year-olds. It always surprises me because I really do not see age. Funny thing is my students are some of the strongest people I know!

If we are going to live well into our nineties or later, we cannot start labelling sixty or sixty-five as being 'old.' I prefer to look at our retirement years as the time for us to redefine ourselves and our lives. We spend most of our younger years working, serving and caring for others. In our sixties, we can turn this around and rediscover who we are and decide where we want to go and who we want to become. How exciting!

I had a gentleman come up to me today at the gym and tell me that he is 'old' before he even told me his name. I only see potential when you approach me. I do not judge you based on your age. I will do my best to keep you safe and you must promise me that you will stop calling yourself, 'old.' Hold your head high. You're in class getting stronger, preparing for the best years of your life. Let's stay positive and work together to change stereotypes.

# STRESS AND THE CONNECTION TO ALZHEIMER'S?

May 19, 2016

Yesterday, I was reading through some old Oprah magazines that I had collected as a subscriber. Some people collect National Geographic, I happened to be into Oprah. The fun thing is that I now have time to read but when I was subscribing, I was lucky to catch an article here and there. I am glad that I have not thrown them out yet. I came across this article from the July 2014 issue, "Fuzzy Life, Fuzzy Brain?" by Laura Hilgers. This article explored the possible links between midlife stress and the development of dementia.

"The researchers had tracked 800 women in Gothenburg, Sweden, from 1968 to 2005, looking at how stress affected their health pre- and post-menopause." They discovered that those who had experienced serious stress as a result of divorce, job loss or death of a spouse around the ages of 38 and 54 "had a 21 percent increased risk of Alzheimer's and a 15 percent increased risk of developing any kind of dementia. The more stressors, the higher the risk." (Hilgers, 2014, The Oprah Magazine, p.62.)

We already know that constantly living under stressful conditions affects our health negatively. Hilgers explains that the hormones that are released to help our body handle stress are meant to be there for short term survival, i.e.to help us escape danger. When these hormones are constantly present, they start to negatively affect neurons and their ability to function properly which can result in cognitive decline.

This article went on to suggest that we need to do all we can on a daily basis to relieve our stress. Hilgers says that research "indicates that if we make a conscious effort to calm down after a traumatic event with a range of stress reduction techniques-cognitive-behavioral therapy, regular exercise, strong social support and mindfulness activities like yoga and meditation-we may help prevent further neural damage." (Hilgers, 2014, The Oprah Magazine, p 63.)

Yet another good reason to try a yoga class because who has not experienced stress at midlife?

Better to be safe than sorry. Reach out if you would like some help with this.

Beth

# SPORT PSYCHOLOGY

October 29, 2015

In the September/October issue of Canfitpro Magazine, Dr. Hayley Perlus has written an article entitled, "Mental Toughness Training for Endurance Athletes." I do not work with endurance athletes who are running marathons but I do work with students well into their late seventies and early eighties and to me these two groups of people have many things in common. 'Working out' for the older crowd is about going the distance and staying fit right up until life's finishing line. We are all on a race course of sorts; the race course of life. As Dr. Perlus points out, the challenges faced by her clientele are threefold: pain, intensity and fear. Seniors face these obstacles every day just in a different form. Her suggestion is that it is how we handle each of these challenges that determines our success.

My students taught me many years ago, that most of them live with constant pain in their joints. "Beth, if you wake up one day and you have no pain, it means that you are dead!" That is a direct quote. I have watched all of them show up to class, without exception and push themselves through the exercises. I always caution them to listen to their bodies but what I see is that they have learned to navigate the pain just like an athlete does. Dr. Perlus recommends using visualization to power through. She says to focus on skill mastery which is exactly what my students do. They focus on learning that new dance or those new moves. They distract themselves from the pain in order to keep moving forward!

When teaching I remind my students to keep track of how they are feeling. Dr. Perlus teaches us that proper pacing is the key to success. We do not want to use too much energy too fast and not be able to complete the class. Again my senior students are experts at pacing themselves. The students who are the most successful are the ones who listen to the cues from their bodies. It is all about checking in with your performance regularly. Dr. Perlus wants her athletes to ask themselves, "Does my race feel faster today?" Or, "Am I thinking clearly?" This is excellent advice for anyone. During your workout check in with your performance. Stay focused on how you are doing compared to the last time you were with me and then adjust accordingly.

Fear for the athlete means worrying that you will not make it up the next hill. I would argue that seniors face this type of fear daily, however they face it with a great sense of purpose and humour. Dr. Perlus says that, "Fear makes us retreat while challenges make us defeat." What a great way to view life. She suggests that we must feel our fears but face them anyway. My students have taught me this time and time again. They show up to class to keep the fear from getting in the way of living. Life gets harder and harder as we age because our bodies and lives are changing so unpredictably. It would be easy to stay home and feed into all of our fears about getting to class; the drive, the road conditions, the possibility of accidents etc. The key is to face these fears but to focus on achieving your goal and go to class anyway! The joys will far outweigh the risks.

I bet you have never considered yourself to be an Endurance Athlete. Well to all of my students I say that you are the best athletes I know! I am so proud of all of you!

Beth

# "ANYTHING YOU DON'T USE, YOU WILL LOSE!"

September 25, 2017

Last Wednesday, I had the pleasure of meeting Miranda Esmonde-White at a lecture held in the Pointe Claire Library. Miranda is founder of Essentrics® and author of *Aging Backwards* and *Forever Painless*. For those of you who don't know, Essentrics® is a 'dynamic stretch workout for all fitness levels that tones, shapes and rebalances the entire body.'

I have to say that I'm very excited about this relatively new trend in the industry because of the focus on stretching. I have been teaching fitness for almost twenty years now, and about half way through my career I realized that we were doing a disservice to our clientele by only giving them five minutes of stretching at the end of our classes. So I started to dedicate a minimum of fifteen minutes at the end of each workout to stretching. There was a little bit of grumbling at first mainly because people do not like change but now all of my students look forward to that time!

The truth is we cannot expect our muscles to perform optimally if they are tight. Muscle conditioning in particular is meant to build muscle which can result in tightness if you do not spend enough time stretching after your workouts. We need to be able to move through the full range of motion of each joint or we are at risk for injury. As Miranda said in her lecture, "No one has a free ride." We all need to put in the work so that we can enjoy life to the fullest.

How many of you right now are able to bend forward and touch your toes? How many of you have pain in your knees, back, shoulders and neck? I meet people every single day who are living a limited life because of joint pain. Perhaps the Essentrics®Technique can help you get back on track.

I do agree with Miranda that if 'you do not use it, you will lose it.' Miranda's workout claims to use all 620 muscles in the body 'with exercises that mimic daily life.' In doing this you are telling your body, "Hey, I still need that and don't let that part of me wither away just yet."

In her lecture Miranda stressed that her technique does not give instant results. The movements are done slowly and it is over time that you will begin to see amazing results. I would argue that the same is true for fitness in general. You cannot neglect your body for 20, 30 or 40 years and expect a trainer to fix all of your issues in one week or month!

To be honest, I walked away from that lecture feeling like I am on the right track as a teacher. While Miranda suggests that we stop lifting weights and doing aerobics and even yoga, I believe that moderation and variety is the key. I have always told my clients to vary their exercise routines during the week to incorporate as many different types of exercise as possible to prevent overuse injuries. I recommend that we continue to do the sports that we love safely and add Essentrics® training to our repertoire.

Miranda strongly suggests that you seek out properly certified Essentrics instructors. They are listed on her website: www.essentrics.com. You can purchase instructional DVDs from this site if you would like to try it in the privacy of your own home but Miranda does recommend that you attend a class once in a while to make sure that you are performing the exercises properly.

Get moving! See you soon,

Beth

# EXERCISING HELPS FIGHT OFF DEMENTIA

June 29, 2015

I have been teaching some clients in my group fitness class-es for 18 years. If they started with me when they were 50 years old (when they were eligible to be in the senior's exer-cise program) that means that they are now 68. Some clients began classes with me when they retired, so a few of them are now in their mid-80's.

Thankfully the changes I have seen in their bodies over this time frame have been mainly positive. I like to tell my students that they have frozen time, that they look exactly the same as they did when they started. I really mean this. For the most part, their bodies move and look the same. What I have noticed is a slight decline in cognitive functioning but out of approxi-mately one hundred and twenty students, I have only a handful of clients that I am worried about. I am happy to say that these few students have a wonderful circle of friends that go with them to the gym and keep them going in the right direction, literally. Mainly I am seeing changes in speed. Students who used to be able to process verbal cues quite rapidly, now need a bit more time. This is normal aging. Forgetting our lefts from our rights etc.

"In 2011, 747,000 Canadians were living with cognitive im-pairment, including dementia - 14.9 percent of Canadians 65 and older. By 2031, this figure will increase to 1.4 million." (Can-fitpro Magazine- March/April 2013. *Exercise and Dementia*. Jennifer Salter). In her article, Jennifer goes on to say," Starting at about  age 40, we lose on average five percent of our over-all brain volume per decade, up until age 70, when a variety of different conditions can accelerate the process. Exercise is one of the few ways to counter the process of aging because it slows down the natural decline of the stress threshold. It is actually good for cells to periodically be subjected to mild stress - this improves their ability to cope with more severe stress. In addition, exercise sparks connections and growth among the cellular network of the brain by increasing the blood volume, regulating fuel, and encouraging neuronal activity and neurogenesis (development of new nerve cells). Regular exercise also increases dopamine levels. Dopamine is a neurotransmitter that is the core of the reward and motivation systems - a lack of which causes irritability, depression, and apathy among many older adults."

I am not a doctor but I am on the ground working with people as they age and I have no doubt in my mind that exercise is the key to staying healthy mentally. I believe that there is real benefit in group exercise classes where you have to actually follow a teacher. It is easy to go for a walk or do the same thing that you do all of the time. The benefits happen when you practice using your brain to complete a new set of challenges. Having to move left as a group. Having to raise your left arm one way and your right another. Having to remember simple choreography. All of this keeps you young. I have seen it. I live this every day with my amazing students.

Try a new class today. Encourage some cell growth in your brains. Do something different to keep your listening, and mobility skills, sharp.

See you in class everyone!

Beth

# CAN WE FIGHT OLD AGE?

February 20, 2017

This is definitely a popular question. In fact one student introduced herself to me this session by saying, "Will this class bring my knees back to what they were?" I need to be careful not to make false claims so I told her that if her doctor has insisted that she start exercising, then she is the right place. I'm sure that she wanted to hear a different answer but the truth is every situation is different and I can't guarantee results. What I do know with absolute certainty is that if people commit to coming to class regularly, they will take a big step toward slowing the aging process and everything that entails.

I'm currently taking a course called, *Active Aging*, with canfitpro. In this course, we are learning that after the age of 60-65 there are certain physiological changes that occur regardless of our fitness level. For example, we lose many of our fast twitch motor units. As a result, the remaining units end up serving more fibres, which can mean that we might lose some fine motor control and coordination. I purposely build in exercises to challenge my students' sense of balance, coordination and cognition during every class. I believe that the more we practice and use these skills, the longer we can avoid long term negative changes.

In my opinion, the name of the game after the age of 65 is maintenance through formal fitness. While I cannot promise to return your joints to the condition that they were in years ago, I am certain that if done properly, exercise can rebalance the muscles around the impacted area and help to prevent further damage. My students continue to enjoy their favourite sports in their eighties, so I know there is truth to this statement.

Beth

# HOW WOULD YOU SPEND YOUR LAST DAY?

September 18, 2015

Recently I learned of the passing of one of my students, whom I had not seen regularly in my classes for quite some time. She was only 69 years old and apparently she died from a stroke. I do know that her husband had passed away in February and that these past few months had been very difficult for her. When we learn of a tragedy such as this, it forces us to stop and evaluate our lives. If today was your last day on earth, how would you spend it?

I am asking the question to get you to think about how you are spending your time versus how you would **LOVE** to spend your time. Many of us have to work and we have lots of responsibilities that we have to honor throughout the day, however I am sure that if you discovered you had only so long to live, that you would make adjustments to your schedule if you could. Why do we wait to live fully, when waiting to do the things that we love could result in us never getting the chance to live the way we want to?

In learning of this lady's passing, I woke up this morning thinking that I have to make a few changes to my routine so that I can do more of the things that bring me joy. For instance, when I leave work I rush into a wall of cars and inch along at twenty kilometers an hour for over an hour to make my way home. Starting today, I am going to pick up a lovely snack and head down by the lake. I will get some beach time in while the traffic clears and I will be doing something that I love. This is just a small change but it will result in me feeling happier and more joyful.

I encourage you to make one small, lasting change to your routine today. We have to live fully while we are here. Call an old friend. Find time to laugh so hard that you cry. Breathe deeply and love completely!

Beth

# SHOULD YOU WRITE A MEMOIR?

May 1, 2017

Most of my time is spent teaching fitness but my other passion is reading, writing and most recently, researching my family history. Both of my parents wrote their life story. It is so wonderful to have this to pass down to my kids but truth be told, I was only interested in their memoirs once I was older and now I wish they had left more information.

My parents are deceased now so I am sorry that I cannot ask them all of the questions that I should have asked them while they were alive. I have taken it upon myself to pick up my mother's research concerning some missing pieces in our family tree. The work is both fascinating and frustrating. I have found boxes and boxes of family photos and almost none of them have names or dates written on the back. Unfortunately, this makes the photos useless as no one else in the family knows these people.

If you are planning on writing your memoir, I would suggest starting with that photo box that you probably have stashed away in the closet. When you look at each picture, write the names of the people on the back with an approximate date and before you know it, a story will start to emerge. Even if you just write about the photos, instead of attempting to write a book, your family will appreciate the time you took to keep the memories alive. Believe me!

If you are not interested in writing your life story, just put the photos back into the box and leave it for the next generation to piece together. You will have left them a wonderful gift.

I hope my blog motivates you to work on your own story for future generations.

Beth

# THE EMPTY DRAWER

July 20, 2015

We tend to have one drawer in our house that collects things. Broken items that could one day be fixed. Miscellaneous parts that may one day find their way back to the original piece. I am guilty of having a few of these drawers. Some of them are so full that they are hard to close.

One of my friends (80 years young) recently emptied her junk drawer and took a picture of it. She sent it to her adult children, all living in their own homes, with their own junk drawers. Her email simply said, "You're welcome." If they got it, they did not let on. I believe one of the kids even sent back a question mark, probably wondering if Mom was starting to lose it.

I understood it all too well, having emptied my dad's home where he lived for over thirty years. There were so many junk drawers. So much unfinished business. It took me a full month of hard work to sort it all out. I applauded my friend. I told her how much her kids will thank her if they are not left to make these decisions after she is gone.

My father was so ill during the last year of his life that he was held up in a hospital bed, waiting for a space to open in long term care. He had been told that it was unsafe for him to return to his home. Let that sink in for second. Imagine if after leaving your house in a hurry, you were then told that you could not return and that someone else was now going to have to pack up all of your things and sell your home. What a crazy thought.

Luckily Dad had family to help with this process but even then, I am sure he was cringing knowing everything that he had left unfinished. To ease the process I took pictures of every item my father owned. I catalogued his whole life and together we sat and went through the important things and he decided where he wanted everything of value to go.

In the end, we found a place for everything. Very little went to a landfill. We had a garage sale and gave most of the furniture to stores that could sell it for a small profit. I brought home papers that needed further consideration.

Dad passed away four months after we sold his home. I stared at those boxes of paper for years until last summer. In taking my time, I found many treasures related to our family history that could have been lost forever. My hope is that I will put them in order and give them a place. I guess in the end, these drawers that we all have, are really drawers of 'hope.' We *hope* to get back to them one day and deal with the items properly.

If you won't do it for yourself, clean out a drawer this week for your family and for your own peace of mind.

Have a great day everyone.

Beth

# PART FOUR

# NUTRITION AND DIETING

**A**s a former PRO TRAINER with canfitpro, I was responsible for teaching the next generation of Fitness Instructor Specialists and one of the most important messages that I had to hammer home to my students was that we do not work outside of our certification. Very often trainers are asked to offer nutritional advice because they happen to be in great shape, and we all want to know what they're doing to get those amazingly defined muscles! However, it is important to speak to a registered dietician about any changes that you might want to make to your current diet so that you can avoid health complications. Unless your fit pro is certified to give nutritional consultations, please steer clear of following any free advice until you have checked it with your doctor.

As a Healthy Weight Loss Coach, I am certified to help you meet your nutritional objectives once they have been set by yourself and your dietician. I help my clients to plan ahead for any potential pitfalls that might sabotage their success, but I am not allowed to advise you on anything other than Canada's Food Guide. The Guide was updated in the last two or three years and if you aim to follow that manner of eating you should be able to meet your nutritional needs.

Over the years I have tried to offer sound guidance on a few topics of nutrition, staying completely within my certification and the following section might provide the inspiration you need to start eating better today.

One of the biggest tips that I share freely is the minimum amount of water that you should be consuming per day. Here is the calculation that I use in my coaching. On average a person needs 30 ml of water per day per kilogram of body weight.

Simply do the conversions based on your weight and then aim to meet that minimum requirement. You will be surprised how well you will feel by meeting the goal. I need to drink three full water bottles a day and to achieve this, I put rubber bands around the bottle and remove them as I empty it. Some people reward themselves with something unrelated to food to encourage their water drinking habit. Be creative and watch your health improve through increased hydration.

I hope the following blog posts will help you on your journey!

# BUT HOW DID I GET FAT?

March 31, 2016

I get asked this question all of the time by frustrated clients who honestly do not understand how they gained those annoying extra pounds.

In their book, *Thinner This Year*, Chris Crowley and Jen Sacheck, explain how it is usually tiny dietary changes that result in those extra pounds. Just like Rome was not built in a day, the pounds get added gradually until one day we realize that our clothes are not fitting properly.

Chris and Jen use the following example to help us understand what can happen. Let's assume that you were in perfect shape and that you were at your ideal weight when you were in your twenties. Yes, you ate well but you also burned each calorie that you consumed. You were in balance. Now let's assume that you add just 10 calories a day to your diet but do not work out more to burn them off. It does not seem significant but that small change will result in one pound of weight gain in a year. If you keep doing this for ten years, you will have gained ten pounds. If you keep doing this for another ten years, you will have gained twenty pounds. So now you are in your forties and you have gained twenty pounds and you have no idea how this happened because the tiny changes in your diet seemed insignificant.

Another problem is that our metabolism slows down as we age, so if we are not careful with our food choices then that innocent looking cookie or that small bag of chips or that extra glass of wine will add up. The good news is that it works in the reverse as well. If we exercise every day and eat less, we will lose those pounds. I am not saying that it's easy but I have seen it happen time and time again.

You must be very honest with yourself. Look at the calories that you are drinking and eating. If you want to make a change, you know what you have to do. Change how you are eating and move more. Get your butt off that chair and into a class. Being with other people can motivate you to stay on track.

Hope this helps.

Beth

# SPORT NUTRITION TIPS – THREE IMPORTANT QUESTIONS TO ASK YOURSELF

October 22, 2020

Yesterday, I had the pleasure of hosting a lecture over Zoom on sport nutrition with registered Dietician and Nutritionist, Marie-Hélène Bourbonnais. My Virtual Fitness Studio students loved Marie-Hélène's energy and practical advice.

I often get questions like: "What foods should I eat just before a class, and when should I eat so I don't feel sick during the class?"

Marie-Hélène shared some very valuable tips and she did so by asking us to consider three important questions first.

1. Does the snack or meal contain fiber?
2. Can the snack or meal be a liquid?
3. How much space will the food in question take up in my stomach?

Marie-Hélène explained that while it is important to eat a variety of carbohydrates, proteins and healthy fats, which will give us energy and the mental focus that we need to exercise safely, we need to be careful about when we are eating them in relation to the workout time.

For example, one hour before a class she wants us to select carbohydrates that will digest quickly and provide energy, keeping in mind the three questions above. The more fibre and fat that there is in the food, the longer it will take to digest, which could result in stomach upset. Drinking the food, such as a smoothie will digest faster so this is a good option, but we need to consider how much we are taking in as well.

She recommends keeping a notepad nearby and tracking our digestive experience. Did we have more energy during the workout with this particular food in our diet? Or did we feel sluggish. The important note here is you need to do what works for you and you can only discover this through trial and error.

Marie-Hélène made it clear that we need to eat before a class, so that we have energy. Remember that your body has depleted its energy stores all night while you were sleeping. In the morning we need to replenish our system with water and food but we need to be mindful of how close to exercise that we are eating.

Protein is important in our diet however Marie-Hélène made it clear that protein takes long to digest so it should only be eaten well in advance of a workout. She recommends that two hours before a class we eat a combination of protein and carbohydrates. Fiber and protein are important in our diet but if we eat our eggs and yogurt and whole wheat toast too close to class, our body will have to work hard digesting while we are exercising. This may leave us feeling sluggish and deprive us of energy. I am guilty of eating a big breakfast an hour before class now that I work from home. I learned a very important lesson yesterday.

Thirty minutes before a workout Marie-Hélène suggests that we only take in liquid nutrients, but again everyone is different and we need to experiment to discover what is right for us. Coffee and tea are fine but caffeine is also a laxative, as she explained, so we have to be careful how close to class we enjoy our beverages. The same goes for water. Ideally three cups of water, two hours or more before class will help our workout but drop that to one cup, thirty minutes before class so have less in our stomach and bladder!

Marie-Hélène will return in the New Year to discuss what we should be eating after our workouts to repair and prepare the body for the next session!

I hope these tips help you to plan your meals accordingly so that you can perform optimally in class.

Beth

# NUTRITIONAL GUIDANCE FROM A DIETICIAN

October 14, 2020

To the members of my Virtual Fitness Studio, I offer free lectures given by top experts on various topics within the field of exercise science and well being. Last week, dietician and international speaker, Tricia Silverman, spoke to us about nutrition and she gave us many valuable tips on everything from reading food labels to calorie counting. Her advice was general and she made it clear that we should seek the advice of a dietician if we are looking for strategies more tailored to our specific situation.

One of the biggest takeaways that resonated with me is that we should be eating three fruits a day of different colours. I started practicing this the very next day. Tricia also recommends that we eat fish twice a week and those varieties that are typically low in mercury such as salmon.

Calorie counting is indeed important for weight loss and Tricia suggests that if we cannot seek the advice of a registered dietician, that we use a BMR calculator which will help to determine the minimum amount of calories that your body needs to function at rest. Armed with this information you need to also take into account your activity level and obviously adjust the calories accordingly.

One of the problems that can arise when we stop exercising for a few weeks or a month, is that we forget to eat less and before you know it, we have gained weight. Tricia taught us that 110 extra calories a day can equal ten pounds a year in weight gain. Please seek help if you are looking to lose weight by restricting your calorie intake.

Tricia suggests that we also take a look at the food label of anything we are about to buy and look for food that is low in sodium, low in sugar and low in saturated fat. Ultimately, we want to eat foods that are high in fiber, as this will help us to feel full longer, resulting in fewer calories consumed. We also learned that when it comes to the listed percentages on the labels, 5% is less and 15% is high.

Tricia told us that her favourite protein sources are fish, beans, chicken and turkey. She wants us to limit our intake of red meat and she advises that we be careful with how many eggs we are eating because it can raise our LDL (lousy) cholesterol. Tricia mentioned that she likes Greek yogurt and pumpkin seeds for protein as well.

Tricia highlighted the negative effects that added sugars have on our body and recommends that we stop drinking pop because sugar is too easy to overconsume when it is in liquid form. When it comes to butter or margarine, she would prefer that we stick to small amounts of butter or extra virgin olive oil. One image that I will never forget from her slide show was the one that depicted the amount of fat in one poutine. It equals three sticks of butter!

And finally Tricia showed us how using smaller plates can help us to lose weight. She showed us half a cup of cooked rice on two different sizes of plates. On the small plate, it looked like we were getting more which in the end can help us to feel less deprived. Opt for smaller plates and then she suggests the 80% rule. Don't eat until you are stuffed but only 80% full.

I hope that some of these facts help you on your journey towards optimal health!

Beth

# WHAT ARE YOU EATING?

April 29, 2015

My question to you today is: what are you eating to fuel you throughout your day?

I meet hard working people every day in the gym. People who show up daily, do the exercises I have prescribed and still they cannot seem to lose those last ten to fifteen pounds. If this sounds like your story, you are not alone. I am going to let you in on a secret. What you eat is more important than what you do at the gym. Let me repeat this. What you **Eat**, is more important than what you do with me at the gym. Some of you will be reminding me of this when we are getting ready to do our sit-ups tomorrow! You still need to exercise, I promise you that but you also need to think about how you are fuelling those workouts.

People can get very upset when I start to inquire about what they are eating, however, if you are telling me that you have literally tried everything to lose weight, then we need to take an honest look at your diet. The good news is you can shed the pounds simply by making simple changes.

I have spent the last year totally changing my diet. I now eat far more than I ever did before and I weigh ten pounds less. This is because I am making far healthier choices. I eat lots of protein and tons of vegetables and fruit. I drink only one small cup of coffee a day with almond milk and the rest is water! And yes, I eat pie and cookies (gluten- and lactose-free.)

The answer really is simple. Move more and eat better. Avoid added sugars in all of the food you eat. Drink water! This is all much easier than coming to see me. I still want you to be in my classes of course but examining what you are eating and how it may be sabotaging your efforts is a great place to start.

# "THREE FOOD INTERFERENCE"-J.D

September 18, 2017

I'm a big fan of Julie Daniluk and her books, *Slimming Meals That Heal* and *Meals That Heal Inflammation*. Julie is a Registered Holistic Nutritionist (RHN) and a leading nutritionist who often appears on the Marilyn Denis Show. I first saw her there and was so impressed with her enthusiasm,that I picked up her books to help me deal with my gluten allergy. That was years ago and I'm happy to say that Julie's recipes helped me to heal my skin. Many of you have seen me drinking her 'Hazelnutty Hot Chocolate' before exercise class. Well, that recipe is found in *Slimming Meals That Heal* and it gives me the energy that I need to get through my fitness filled days.

I'm currently watching a free video series that Julie has started to help people heal inflammation in their bodies, which might be the cause of sore joints, bloating, headaches etc. In yesterday's video she told us about the 3 Food Interference tactic. Many of us reach for sweets or chips or other treats when we feel we need a boost or a reward. Giving into these cravings can make us feel great in the moment but over time lead to unwanted weight gain. Julie suggests that before we give into the craving "We stare down the food and then put three healthy foods in front of it." She wants us to eat one protein, one healthy fat and one fibrous food so that we will feel full before we dig into the treat and therefore, we will eat less of the food that isn't good for us. This is brilliant and I plan on putting this tactic into action, however it will take some planning to make sure that the good food is readily available. I encourage you to pick up one of her books today.

Beth

# "I'M HAPPIER BEING FAT!"

November 2, 2015

Those were her words, not mine, as Lady X, a newly acquired friend of mine wolfed down her second piece of pie. She looked at me sideways as I sat there drining my water and asked me if I ever eat dessert. If you know me, you know that I do not hold back on food, especially dessert! I used to make wedding cakes and birthday cakes for money as a part time business and that involves a real passion for both baking and eating! In all fairness though, it takes a bit less to fill me up so I often get accused of restricting my diet.

For some reason, people who barely know me, feel the need to confess to me their dietary sins. On many occasions people have become quite defensive about their food choices and lifestyle with absolutely no provocation from me whatsoever. "Oh, you are a trainer? Well let me tell you...."

Most of the time I can wiggle out of the conversation and direct it in the appropriate direction. On this particular visit with Lady X however, it seemed to be her mission to prove to me that even though I had not asked about her happiness level or even her weight, she was indeed a much happier person being fat.

I do not judge people as being fat or thin. I look at the overall picture of a person but this individual was carrying a dangerous amount of weight around her middle, she herself would have no problem telling you this. To be clear, we were meeting about something entirely unrelated to fitness and weight loss.

I did manage to put the conversation back onto the subject at hand but I did not really address her beliefs that losing the weight made her miserable. Her position is not unique. I have heard it before from other people who feel that it sucks to eat a healthy diet. These people maintain that there is no joy in eating salad. I am laughing as I write this because it always takes me by surprise. It is funny how we now associate happiness with the pleasure we derive from physically eating our food. Instead of eating for nourishment, it is all about the experience of eating.

I would argue that if you feel like Lady X, that it is not the weight around your middle that is making you unhappy. Something much deeper is causing you to feel down or sad and those feelings that you are avoiding is the reason that you are reaching for the dessert or whatever vice you have chosen to push the emotions aside. It is the ultimate game of distraction. "Oh I feel sad about....oooo look, pecan pie!"

People have to be ready to deal with the emotional baggage that causes us to overeat and overindulge. As a trainer, I can put you on a program and I can help you to lose the weight but only if you are 100% on board with healing yourself inside and out. The choice is yours.

Take steps today toward developing a total care plan for yourself. This can be as simple as heading to the bookstore and picking up a book. Maybe you can join a meditation class. The step need not be huge. I have told you before that you have to nourish the mind, the body and the soul. It is all related. When one area is out of balance you need to face it head on to make lasting changes in your health.

Beth

# WANT TO LOSE TEN POUNDS?

July 10, 2015

Yesterday, Dr Oz had a segment on his show that highlighted an overweight woman who was consuming many sodas a day. As part of her effort to become healthier, she stopped drinking sodas and lost ten pounds in one week. I know that this is possible as this happened with a client of mine whom I was personally training in 2007.

Her name was Linda. She was in her 50s and she wanted to get healthier and lose weight. She was 5'4" and she weighed 169 pounds. She just wanted to lose ten pounds to start. During the interview, she told me what her daily food intake looked like. She was consuming two litres of Diet Coke or Pepsi a day! I suggested that simply taking that habit out of her routine would result in weight loss. Linda looked me right in the eye and told me that she "would never stop drinking her sodas as that was it too important to her." I proposed that we simply get moving more and discuss her diet later when the exercise was going well.

To my surprise she arrived a week later full of smiles. She had given up the soda and lost ten pounds! I trained her from September to December and by December 1st she had lost 22 pounds and she looked amazing. What a great Christmas present.

If you want to lose weight and you drink soda, even diet soda, give it up for two weeks and see how your life will change. Replace it with water or herbal tea. Start moving more and you will see results.

Beth

# SOCIALIZING AND GLUTEN INTOLERANCE

October 1, 2015

It has been almost a year since I finally made the connection between my symptoms and gluten. My life and health have improved so much over this past year. I have to say though that the hardest part remains socializing with others over meals. 'Breaking bread' together is so often how we choose to visit with friends and family.

People try so hard to be helpful and make menu suggestions that would appear to be safe for me but really they are not because the kitchen in which the food is prepared has to be a gluten-free environment from the start. Many loved ones are so convinced that they can cure me and that their food is safe that I have often folded under the pressure and eaten things that I know are not good for me, to put an end to the conversation.

When you go to a party or sit with friends, you want to forget your troubles and most of all you do not want to have to educate others about the gravity of the situation. When I showed some of my family some photos that I took of my skin in a flareup, they finally understood how serious this is for me but really it should not have to get to that point.

If you are around someone who is struggling with a dietary restriction, the best thing that you can do is to ask them how they would like to have a visit. Maybe it will be over tea and not lunch or dinner. Maybe they will suggest a restaurant that is safe for everyone or perhaps they will want to bring their own food. Do not be offended if they explain that they cannot eat your food. In my case this is not a matter of being picky. Celiac and dermatitis herpetiformis are awful conditions and we are just doing our best to function in a society that is all about food!

Beth

# THE SOLUTION IS EASY

September 28, 2015

Sometimes I wish that I had a magic pill or an ancient remedy that I could share with everyone to help them lose weight and be healthier. The reason I say this is that people generally do not believe me when I tell them that the answer to their weight loss is within reach, if they make a series of lifestyle changes. People seem to want to believe that those green coffee beans are what they need or that they have to get their hands on the latest, greatest supplement.

People want to believe this because they want to keep living their lives in exactly the same way and be able to lose the weight around their mid-section. People want me to give them exercises but they do not want me to look at what they are actually consuming because it may mean that they have to give up their favourite food, which incidentally may be the reason that they cannot lose weight.

I have had clients tell me directly that they will do all of the exercises I suggest but they will not stop drinking diet soda, nor will they stop eating bread or sugar. One client told me that she hates water. How can someone hate water? What that tells me is that this person has become addicted to sweetened beverages or sugar in general. In my experience, just getting people to stop drinking sweetened beverages and replace all of them with plain water, makes a huge difference in their waist line.

Aside from what people are eating, I tell them to make sure that they are getting formal exercise in every single day. Then the excuses start. "Well I have no time." In my experience, I can find thirty minutes to an hour of idle time in almost everyone's day. Most people are watching television or surfing the net at some point to relax. Swap out that time for a walk or some muscle conditioning and stretching. If there really is no time wasted on watching television etc., then I tell people to get up thirty minutes earlier and do a home-based workout. "But I cannot do that!"

The solution is simple. The problem is you need to get out of your own way!

If you really want to lose weight, that should become your focus until you achieve success. Enlist the help of every professional you can find. Ask your friends to help you by working out together. Shed the house of all processed food (I had to do this because of an allergy and everyone is healthier as a result) and get your family cooking and eating well as a unit. Stop eating out. Drink plenty of water. Avoid all soda and processed sugar. Focus on eating tons of fruit and vegetables and lean protein.

I had no choice but to stop eating almost all processed foods because of an allergy to gluten. While I do not suggest that people follow my diet, I will tell you that not being able to eat bread (I really have not found a yummy replacement) forced me to turn to vegetables and fruits more. The problem may not be the bread but the fact that you are not consuming enough of the other good food groups because you are filling up on bread, crackers, cookies and muffins.

I lost ten pounds within two months simply by changing my diet and I was not looking to lose weight. I lost the weight around my middle. I had resigned myself to the frump of old age but my gluten allergy helped me to become far healthier and now happier.

I know that you wish I had a magic pill but just think how much that pill would cost and invest in the services of a dietician and, if needed, a personal trainer instead!

Beth

# PART FIVE

# FEEL GOOD POSTS

The truth is I am incredibly lucky that people entrust me with their health and fitness. Helping others lifts my spirit and brings me great joy and I do my best to share this with my students.

As the world battles the Corona Virus Disease (COVID-19) pandemic, I am so grateful that my work has continued via a virtual platform and that my students were willing to learn a new skill in order to keep fit over this last year. I am among those who are now able to make a living from the safety of home and I am incredibly grateful for this blessing. I actually believe that all of my training up to this point has prepared me for this unique situation. As a student, I was very familiar with online learning as I have taken many virtual courses on publishing and writing workshops with individuals from all over the world. Though I was a bit nervous at first to try leading fitness through a computer screen, I found my flow rapidly and have been able to keep 100+ seniors fit during lockdown.

Anyone who knows me knows that I do my best to remain positive in the face of adversity so that I can help my students overcome their physical and emotional challenges. I write gratitude lists weekly, if not daily, which helps me to see the glass half full instead of half empty. Most of the time we just need to think outside of the box to remain fit. Life is going to get in the way, but the key is to remain positive and look for opportunities for movement, no matter the circumstance. While it might not be perfect or exactly what you are used to, joy can be found with the right attitude.

I hope that you will enjoy these 'feel good' posts.

# WITH ALL MY HEART

April 30, 2015

I had to take a picture of myself yesterday after class, as half-way through the cardio segment, as I was working up quite the sweat, a heart appeared on my chest. I guess I really put my heart into that workout!

Today's message is just a reminder to put your heart into every effort you are making to take care of yourself. Yes, some days are easier than others but I try to remind my students that we are so lucky/blessed, to have this time together. It is a luxury.

When taking care of my dying father a few years back, I spent so much of my time in the hospital. For years, my time was not my own. Unfortunately, we often only realize how good something is, when we lose it. Every moment that we spend in good health, doing what we want to do, when we want to do it, needs to be treasured. I tell my students that they should be smiling from ear to ear because they are able to move and get out and socialize, laugh and play. We take this for granted. Walk, run, dance! Whatever you do, give it your all.

Be fully present in the next yoga class. Be fully present when muscle conditioning or doing your cardio. Do not watch or listen to the news while working out. Try to focus on what you are doing. You will get more out of your efforts that way. Give yourself a gift. The gift of taking care of your heart, mind and body.

With all of my heart, I wish you a fabulous day!

Beth

# YOU HAVE TAUGHT ME SO MUCH

March 8, 2017

Many of you have been in my classes for the last fifteen or eighteen years and as a result you've seen me grow older! I had young children ages two, four and six when I first started teaching. Now they are all adults with lives of their own. I was a very different person back then. I was working three jobs; two in the fitness business and one in an office setting.

Over the years, you have been very supportive and interested in my busy life. You have listened and laughed and commiserated during my years of raising teenagers. When my mother died unexpectedly ten years ago, many of you filled a deep void with your wisdom. You watched me burn the candle at both ends taking care of my ailing father for a year. A number of you took the time to attend my dad's funeral in 2011. I was very touched considering the distance that you had to travel. You have listened to my worries and offered helpful advice and for that I cannot thank you enough. Through all our times together, you have taught me many valuable lessons.

I consider the most important of these to be that we must always keep moving even when life gives us serious challenges. There may be times when our bodies are hurting but there is always something we can do to keep active. The fact that you are still in my classes is proof that moving is the key to lasting health.

Through your example, I have learned that it is important to speak up and be heard, and that it's necessary to do what is in our own best interest. Basically, "if something doesn't feel right, don't do it!"

You have showed me that being kind is more important than being right. While it is important to speak our minds, it's more important to be careful with our words, and sometimes we simply need to walk away from a difficult situation for our own sanity.

You have taught me that we never really know what someone is struggling with and therefore we must tread lightly when approaching others. If someone has been rude to me, it's usually because they are carrying a burden far bigger than I could bear. We must always take the time to listen and understand before we react.

Thank you so much for all that you have shared with me. Your personal stories are inspirational and you keep me going.

Beth

# EMBRACE CHANGE

May 12, 2015

"To be fully alive, fully human, and completely awake is to be continually thrown out of the nest." – Pema Chodron. This is one of my favourite quotes and it is so appropriate with the recent celebration of Mother's Day.

Stress and unhappiness show up in our lives, when we are constantly trying to keep things in our lives the same. The only constant is constant change. The seasons change (if you live in Canada, you are saying "thank God,") our babies become adults and we grow older. Things are constantly moving despite our attempts to nail stuff down and keep everything 'perfect.'

If you were at the gym with me yesterday, you know that we have been thrown out of our 'nest.' They are replacing the roof that has been leaking for many years. We have all been complaining about this and finally it is being fixed but in order for that to happen, we were tossed out of our routine, our comfort zone, our nest.

I love watching people's reaction to change.

Some people are so flexible, others allow themselves to be upset. Our reactions to any event in our lives, are an indication to how we are feeling inside. Does our blood pressure get dangerously high? Do we get chest pains? Do we reach for junk food or alcohol to self soothe? Learning how to deal with the stress of change can help us to improve our health.

If all that you had planned is no longer accessible and you must start over again, what is your first reaction? Do you swear? Do you become angry at the world for once again "letting you down?" Do you consider your day ruined and carry it with you all day, talking about it with anyone who will listen? Or do you laugh and get on with living, using all of the skills you have, to make everyone's day around you, the best that it can be?

This book by Pema Chondron is a wonderful addition to any library. I bought it when my life was in disarray and it really helped me to get through some difficult times. I was working so hard to create the perfect life, when suddenly I had become the main caregiver of my father. I grew very depressed at having to give up all of my plans. Pema's book taught me to learn to embrace change and find joy there!

Use your unique set of skills to transform any situation into a positive experience.

Beth

# MAKE THE WORLD A BETTER PLACE

May 21, 2015

My backyard is filled with trilliums at this time of year and I was moved recently by the sight of one purple flower amongst all of the white ones and it got my thinking. I truly believe that we have it all wrong, when we work so hard to be just like everyone else. We tend to want to look the same, dress the same and speak the same. At times, we may want to blend into the crowd and remain anonymous.

I was very shy as a child and in many ways I still am, though I may not look shy while I'm leading a class! However, when the music is on, I am the happiest I can be, either leading dances or teaching fitness. Suddenly any fears I have about public speaking or making mistakes, vanish and I am comfortable and at ease. My love of music and dance set me apart from the crowd and I'm so happy that I pursued this uniqueness.

This purple flower, growing amongst all of the standard white trilliums stands up and says, "Look at me. I am different in many wonderful ways and yet similar all the same." I believe that we are supposed to celebrate what makes us different and use those gifts to strengthen the ties between us.

In the last few years, I have learned that my success is not going to be in trying to imitate someone else. I have been educated in what I do. I have been in the field working with clients for 17 years. I know what works and what doesn't. In deciding not to follow the crowd, I have found personal strength and immeasurable happiness.

Perhaps I am feeling this way as I get older. I am 48. I have wrinkles. I will not try to wipe them away. I have had three beautiful kids, naturally, therefore I am never going to have that per-fect, pre-baby body (whatever that is?) I spend all morning at the gym, helping others to be the best that they can be and this gives me incredible joy. I get to dance and work with music and get paid for having fun!

How do you recognize your gifts? You will find those gifts in what makes you happiest. Taking part in a favourite sport, reading, writing, singing, dancing, cooking etc. Perhaps you can find a way to share this joy with friends and family. Life is meant to be lived and celebrated. Celebrate the fact that you are original and use your uniqueness to make the world a bet-ter place.

Beth

# EVERYONE IS FIGHTING A BATTLE!

September 24, 2015

Last week, I had the pleasure of meeting many new students into my fitness classes.

One meeting in particular has reminded me that no matter how we look on the outside, all of us are fighting some sort of battle and because of this, we should never judge anyone before we get to know them.

A lovely lady, who I am guessing has passed the young age of 75, participated quietly in my class on the first day. She stood out to me because she reminded me of my mother who passed away eight years ago. She has beautiful blue eyes, bright red lips and freckles and the warmest smile that you can imagine.

On the second day, she came right up to me to tell me that while she loved my class, she could not continue for the next month.  When I asked why, she told me that the hospital had called and that she had to go in for extensive treatments. The details do not matter. What struck me was her mood. I expressed my concern for her situation and wished her well. She then asked me if I had a DVD that she could buy and follow while away from class. I told her that I had been working on one for years but had not finalized this project because I was too busy working. I told her that during this time, she should be thinking about recovering and not working out. With a big bright smile, she said, "Oh, I am not the least bit worried about my health but I think that it is time you got a DVD together don't you?"

I laughed because now not only did she look like my mom, but she sounded just like her as well!

My mother suffered from a number of health problems. Shortly before she died she had lost vision in one eye. She asked me to take her to the eye doctor and when we got there he chastised us for coming, told my mother that she would never see again out of that eye and said that she should have gone directly to the hospital when it had first happened two days prior. My mother was not the least bit fazed. I was freaking out, texting my siblings, and all my mother wanted to do was to go and have potato soup at La Baton Rouge restaurant.

No matter what we look like on the outside, we all are struggling with some sort of situation. We therefore all need to be treated with respect, kindness and love. My mom is the perfect example of someone who did not show her struggles on the outside. We can all smile and get through the day but just because we seem to have life all under control, we can never assume what life is like for anyone.

Beth

# SPEAK YOUR TRUTH

November 16, 2015

A colleague of mine recently told me how impressed she was with the way that I handled a difficult situation. All of my life I have been worried what others will think of me if I say "no," and as a result, I used to say "yes," to everything even when it would make me sad or miserable. Now I make sure that if something does not feel right, I listen to my heart and I speak my truth as soon as it is appropriate.

I do this to keep stress from piling up in my life. I do this to keep healthy. Unspoken words have a way of piling up and weighing us down. I can bet that if you are feeling stressed or unhappy right now it may be linked to some unspoken words or the fact that you are living your life for others, instead of for yourself. This can apply to the work that we are doing or the relationships that we are in. Staying silent when we have so much to say, can make us sick. When you take the time to deal with issues as they come up, it becomes easier to speak your truth and to walk in it.

Watching me navigate this touchy situation impressed my colleague and it seemed to encourage her to do the same. Funny thing is, it happened easily to the point where I did not really even notice that it had happened. I am getting better and better at living my life the way that feels right to me. The first time you present an opposing point of view or the first time that you disappoint someone by refusing to do what they are asking, is the hardest. After that, practice makes perfect!

Remember to make your decisions based on what you value in your life and as much as possible try to walk through this life living your truth. There really is no other way.

Beth

# FOLLOW YOUR HEART

July 23, 2015

"For when the heart goes before like a lamp and illumines the pathway, many things are made clear that else lie hidden in darkness." - Longfellow

I wear my heart on my sleeve (or shirt as in one of my prior blog posts). At times, this has caused me pain but more often than not I have been led to meet wonderful people or have positive experiences. The times that have been disappointing were the occasions where I trusted someone who ended up being completely interested in their own agenda. If I am completely honest with myself and if I put down my ego for a second, I can admit that I did not follow my first instinct in these cases. I was probably motivated by greed or power of some kind. Why else would I let my survival instinct be blurred? We sometimes get dazzled by promises.

I have followed my heart in my career choice. I look around me sometimes and smile, wondering how it is that I get to have so much fun at work! I love helping and teaching. I cannot imagine doing anything else.

As for my marriage, I knew as soon as I met Peter that he was the one I was going to marry. It took him a bit longer to figure this out but eventually we knew from dating other people that we really were a suitable match. Often how we feel is the only indication we get, as to whether we should or should not follow a path. You must follow your heart to find happiness in all aspects of your life.

Beth

# "REST AND BE THANKFUL"

May 18, 2015

"Rest and be thankful." – William Wordsworth.

I am sure that you have heard about the power of gratitude and how focusing on the good things in your life can change your perspective and make you happier. I have known my hus-band Peter for almost 30 years and I swear he was born this way! He is, by far, the happiest person I know.

Many years ago, while working on our home, I came outside to find Peter lying in the wheelbarrow, taking a break. He was so happy to be resting his legs! He tried to convince me to climb in, by telling me how comfortable he was, but on this particular occasion I chose to take a picture instead.

Often, if there is a good song on the radio in his car when he arrives home, he will pull up to the front door, music blasting and insist I come out and sit for a bit and listen. Doesn't matter if I am doing the dishes or writing or cooking, I have to stop what I am doing and take a few minutes to surround myself with his joy! It always has a positive affect on my mood.

If the stars are visible one evening, he grabs my hand and gets me to come outside. He turns all of the house lights off and together we sit and appreciate the view. Nothing like country living to really see the beauty of the night sky! Interest-ing bugs, rainbows, bird songs, you name it, Peter and I have stopped and paused to appreciate.

Moments like this are too numerous to recount. Suffice it to say that because of Peter, I am a much happier person. I begin and end every day thinking of three things I am truly grateful for about my life.

I have been doing this for over three years. It is amazing the transformation that happens in your heart and health when you choose to focus on the good things, instead of all of the dreaded tasks you have to undertake in the day ahead or all of the things that went wrong in the previous twelve hours.

Will you join me in this?

As you sit here, think of three things that bring you joy.

One at a time, think of them, close your eyes and put a little 'Mona Lisa' smile on your face as you take in the good feeling of those things.  Breathe in the joy and suddenly you will feel lighter and brighter and happier!

Beth

# MISTAKES AS TUITION?

July 15, 2015

I recently rushed into something without sleeping on it and it ended up costing me $100. As we are not rich, I was feeling badly about this. My husband is very forgiving and never complains when each of us takes our turn at making mistakes, however I could not shake this sadness.

It really does pay to talk to people (friends) when you are struggling with something. I am quite close to many of my students as they have watched me grow over the years and it is hard for me to hide my emotions. They all know me so well so I decided to share my story with Laura after class and she completely put my mind at ease.

"Beth you have to look at the money you spent as tuition! You learned something from the experience and will never do it again."

Wow, I was so blown away by this statement and I instantly felt better. I spend money every year on staying certified by taking courses and exams, and with a simple change in thinking, I can judge what happened to me as a huge lesson learned.

I need to listen to my gut instinct at all times. I should have gone home and thought long and hard about the purchase before I jumped in. I normally collect information and then study my options. Unfortunately I felt a bit pressured to buy, not necessarily by the seller but because we have a bit of a relationship, I felt I needed to lend my support. Once I got home and researched the product, I instantly knew it was not for me. Lesson learned.

Beth

# WHAT WOULD YOU TELL YOUR FIVE-YEAR-OLD SELF TODAY?

June 19, 2015

I was incredibly shy and filled with insecurity as a young girl so it is ironic that I ended up becoming a personal trainer/fitness instructor, when gym class was my biggest nightmare. No one wanted me on their team because I wasn't good at any of the sports. I hated public speaking and I hated being up at the front of the class! I can attribute my career choice to being supported by good teachers.

After having my first son, I wanted to lose the baby weight so I joined a gym near my mother's home. I would then drop off my son and go there for an hour. I had never taken any fitness classes before. I absolutely loved the positivity of the aerobics teacher. She was engaging and friendly and she made the exercise fun. It was one hour that I could spend on me, two times per week. From there I enjoyed it so much, that after my third child, I went to night school to become a fitness instructor. Looking back on my shy, non-physical five-year-old self, I would now say:

"Keep your chin up Beth, because soon you will be able to do all of the things that you feel so insecure about. Yes, for now you may be the last person picked in gym class however in a few years you will be the one laughing as you get paid well to help your students to do push-ups, sit-ups and lunges. Your classes will be filled to capacity because your students will feel inspired and motivated to be the best that they can be under your guidance. You will change lives for the better."

Find an old picture of yourself today and ask yourself, "What would you say to that little girl or boy looking back at you?"

Realize how far you have come. You have succeeded in getting through some of life's most difficult moments. Even if for just a few moments, celebrate your success and feel good about your accomplishments.

Beth

# PATIENCE OF AN ANGEL

October 31, 2018

This week, as I was heading to my locker in the family changing room, I almost ran into a woman who was coming out of one of the large cabins. We both apologized for the near miss but she did not smile or offer any opening for conversation which is unusual at our gym. I am quite used to having in depth discussions with strangers in our facility but not everyone is there for a chat. I moved my stuff out of her way to give her ample space and then her situation became abundantly clear.

Out of the same cabin where she had just been, a gentleman appeared who looked to be about the same age. I would give them both late sixties or early seventies. He was moving quite slowly and sat down beside her. I watched as she dried his feet and tried to coach him through putting on his socks before his shoes. This was a tiresome task as he was insistent that it was time for him to put on his shoes. I remain in awe at her patience through this whole process. Many of us have had to dress our own kids or grandkids and we know how difficult this can be. Usually kids are much smaller and easy to manage. All I could think about was how much harder this would be if he were physically defiant. He was twice her size.

Once his shoes were tied he sat quietly and watched his caregiver, maybe wife, brush her hair in the mirror. I found this quite touching. I looked away briefly to pick up my bags and as I was passing them I noticed that he had a child's comb in his hands and he was combing his own hair off to one side just like a little boy would do. I can't make any assumptions about his condition but I witnessed immeasurable patience and love and wondered if I myself could be that strong.

I wished them both a wonderful day and each of them smiled in return. They seemed quite surprised that I would speak to them at all!

We must be thankful for the little things in life and remember that being kind is always appreciated, especially by those who bear huge responsibility for the welfare of others. Often just a simple smile will brighten someone's day and in turn this will help them to carry on.

Beth

# DO YOU SEE THE LITTLE THINGS?

June 9, 2015

I guess because we live in the country, my husband and I have a thing for creatures big and small. We have a stream behind our home so we often have dragonflies flying around our garden and backyard. Occasionally they get stuck in one of our carports and instead of letting them die, we save them.

Last week, when I was at the spa resting in one of the solarium areas, I heard the familiar sound of a dragonfly's wings, beating against the window pane. There were people all around not noticing this poor fly trying to get outside. I did not want to cause a scene or disturb people's rest, so I waited until just two people remained in the area. I approached the fly who, by this time, was frantically trying to squeeze himself through what looked like a crack in the wall.

Most people I know would smash him to bits or ignore him altogether and let him die of starvation or exhaustion but not me, I have to make his survival my goal! I do this with spiders in my house if they are small. If they are big I have to get someone braver to pick them up. I really am a bit crazy but I hate destroying life. It makes me feel terrible. If I am teaching and there is a bug on the floor, I get so stressed because now I have make sure I don't accidentally step on him, as I care for all of the students in the room at the same time. What did I tell ya? Crazy.

So as I stood at the spa window digging for him to come out of the crack, people were starting to wonder what the heck I was doing. So I started talking to him. "Come on now, I just want to help, do not make a fool of me. Let's do this together."

Well after a bit of prying, he committed to riding on my finger as I carried him away from the window. I fully expected him to freak out and head back to his hiding spot but he stayed put. In fact, I was able to walk all around outside with him and he would not leave my hand. I tried putting him down several times but he wanted to stay!

At this point, I could feel myself becoming red and a bit embarrassed as I walked around the hot tubs with this big bug on my hand. I was honoured that he trusted me enough to stay so long. I got a chance to take in his colours and beauty for so long. Eventually he agreed to be put down on a plant leaf and we parted ways.

The moral of this story is to listen for the little things in life.

We are so bombarded by loud noises and music and advertising that we often cannot hear the bird singing or a dragonfly's wings flapping. It is quite a sound. Apparently it can fly at 45 mph, it can fly backwards like a hummingbird, it can hover like a helicopter and also it can also fly straight up and down and side to side. From what I have read, the dragonfly symbolizes change and a sense of self realization. It is seen as a symbol of power and agility, prosperity and good luck.

Next time you get the chance, enjoy the presence of this amazing creature. They really are stunning. Look out for the little things around you today. Breathe and take in the view. We can learn a lot about ourselves and others living like this.

Beth

# "WHEN LIFE GIVES YOU LEMONS..."

June 30, 2016

All I could do yesterday was laugh. No point in getting frustrated or upset.

I had prepaid for my gas and then threw my wallet and keys onto the driver's seat. While pumping the gas, my car decided to lock itself. I won't get into what I must have done wrong, as I know that my car has a built in 'lock itself" feature. In all 392,000+ kilometers, this has never been a problem.

I finished pumping the gas but all the while I was considering that I am out in the world 'naked.' No cell phone, no wallet, no keys, just my smile. No big deal. The world is a friendly place. Someone will help me out. Well, it turns out that the gas attendant was having a worse day than I was.

Long story short, and a line up of about six patrons later, she could not find the CAA phone number. So I asked anyone in line if they had CAA because it is written on the back of the membership card. To my surprise, not one person was a member but then none of them offered to 'google' the number for the attendant, to help speed up the process. I was surprised by the lack of desire to help a stranger but I did not let it bother me. Maybe these folks are having a bad day too. Eventually she found the number but then her portable phone would not work. Oh and did I mention I was supposed to be at a doctor's appointment in 20 minutes that I have waited over six months for.

All I could do was laugh. At least it was sunny so I walked to a nearby restaurant for some assistance. The walk was short and pleasant. I would not let this situation get the best of me!

It took me forever to find the manager of the restaurant but he did let me use the phone and he actually 'googled' the CAA number and found it. Then there must have been a new attendant on the phone because it took her much longer than usual to locate me. Again I did not get angry or frustrated. It happens. We all have bad days at work and in life.

CAA was actually there within 30 minutes of locating me and then I watched as this total stranger managed to break into my car effortlessly without any alarm going off. I of course thanked him but wondered secretly about his character. I thought to myself, "Wow what a skill to have. Knowing how to break into any car at any time without the alarm going off."

I was officially ten minutes late for my appointment but over thirty minutes away by car. So I called the office only to find out that they had stopped answering the phone five minutes ago. Everyone was officially on break! Now I was upset but laughing in disbelief. For those of you who live in Quebec you know all too well that we often wait an hour or more to see the doctor once we arrive in the office, so I decided to take a chance and head to the appointment anyway. I had not missed my turn and it all worked out! A happy ending to what otherwise could have been a disastrous story. I really believe that our attitude affects the outcome of our experiences.

I am still laughing and so happy that I stayed the course and did not give up. Still amazed at how easily the CAA man broke into my car...

Beth

# DON'T JUDGE A BOOK...

June 17, 2015

When you look at the front of my home you do not see a manicured lawn. I do not have incredible gardens and a paved driveway with a stone border. I have a very humble house, in a very humble setting. This used to concern me, as I really would worry what the neighbours were saying about our 'lack of a lawn.' A wise person once said to me that "It is none of your business, what other people think of you!"

I try to remember this as I walk through this life. Everyone is entitled to their opinion of you. All that matters is that you live your life, being true to yourself. Part of being true to myself is caring more about my family, my health and my job and less about my lawn. It may be full of weeds but if you look really closely you will see wild strawberries and at this time of year, we often sit in the sun and pick and eat them! They are absolutely delicious!

As my kids were growing up, this was part of the ritual in our area. I gave each of my wee ones a bucket and we went walking around the neighbourhood for berries of all sorts. They grow along the sides of the streets.

I will tell you though that my daughter once collected enough of these tiny berries from our front yard to make a small pie and she was so proud of herself, as it took hours to get that many tiny treasures. So while my life is not about glam and glitter, it is about quality and making lasting memories along the way.

Beth

# THANK THOSE WHO HELPED YOU

June 16, 2015

For those of you who attend my classes, you have heard me speak about Shawna. She currently teaches Physical Education at the college level, however she used to train the teachers coming out of the YMCA Group Fitness Instructor Program. I was one of her students 17 years ago. When I successfully graduated, she gave me my first paying job. Shawna is incredibly supportive to everyone who is lucky to call her 'teacher, boss or friend.'

Shawna shares everything she knows and all materials that she has developed and acquired over the years in order to help all teachers be the best that they can be. Not many teachers/bosses are like this. I have tried as hard as I can to do this in my own work, as I see how important it is for us to be supportive of each other in this industry.

I had the pleasure of attending Shawna's fitness class yesterday as I was on vacation. I felt so happy to be back in her class, even though she decided to put me up front and made me her partner in muscle conditioning! I had no choice but to work hard when really I just wanted to dance and goof off in the background.

We all have those people in our lives who have helped us to become the person we are today. Shawna taught us that as teachers, we don't bring our personal life into the class. We put on a smile no matter what may be going on with us outside of work, as we are being paid to serve and support our clients. She taught us to arrive at least ten minutes before our classes, so that we can get ourselves ready and then have time to chat and get to know our clients.

I can remember her evaluating our aerobic routines as newbie instructors and watching her yell at the teachers who were off the beat. It really did feel like the army.

"You are off...start again. Again. Listen for the beat! Just do it. No..not right. Not good enough.  Fix this!"

We were all scared to death of her I think, but only because we respected her incredible talent so much. She was teaching us to handle pressure and difficult situations so that we would be able to flourish in a real class setting. She wanted us to be successful.

Though she had a tough side, she was extremely funny while sharing her own stories of teaching nightmares and she was always the first one to laugh at anything she may have said or done that was incorrect. She leads with her heart and this is what I love most about Shawna.

Thank you so much for all you have done for me Shawna. I am only successful at teaching fitness because of the time you took to prepare me properly!

My message for today is to reach out to those people who have played a role in making you fabulous and thank them. You will make their day and yours.

Beth

# SWITCH YOUR PERSPECTIVE

July 21, 2015

Just like you, I am dealing with some sort of challenge right now. Some of us are dealing with physical ailments. Some of us are dealing with financial problems. Some of us are struggling in our relationships. My message today is that these challenges can sometimes be disguised as opportunities.

We only get to understand how strong we are when we experience these little setbacks in our lives. If everything were easy, we would not push ourselves to try harder. We would not grow. I believe that the challenge I am facing today is helping me to be a more compassionate person toward others who may be experiencing the same in silence.

We know the signs of someone in distress. Most of us have been there. While the rest of the world rushes by, we can see the sadness in another's eyes and we have the ability to help, simply because we have experienced it ourselves. Perhaps the challenge facing you today is placing you somewhere where you need to be, to help another.

Maybe there is someone who is not as far along on his or her journey as you are and they in fact need you to lend them a hand. Even though we are dealing with very difficult circumstances sometimes, we all still have our skills and if we can use those inherent parts of ourselves to brighten another person's journey, then I believe that our personal struggle will be eased somewhat.

When my father was in the hospital, there were many people who would share the room and then pass on, only to be replaced by a new patient the next day. When you spend a year in the hospital, you see a lot of suffering. I once had the opportunity to talk to an elderly lady who was sharing the room with my father. She was often asleep but on this rare occasion she was awake and in need of help as she had dropped her spoon. As I passed her the spoon, I found something to compliment her on. She had the most beautiful freshly manicured fingernails. Well I made her day by telling her how lovely she looked. She thanked me with tears in her eyes saying that she was alone and was so grateful to have some company.

She died in her sleep that night. I was sad, but happy that I had taken the time to make her smile and glad that I had made her laugh on her last day. This little shift in our perspective, from being a victim to a hero, makes it easier to carry on. I could have turned away and ignored her and continued to focus on the desperation of my personal situation but instead, I allowed my empathetic nature shine through which helped both of us in the end.

Use your ability to make people laugh or your amazing listening skills to help someone out today. You will improve your situation in the process, guaranteed.

Beth

# CONCERN FOR OTHERS

July 3, 2015

As I have mentioned before I love to read about different faith systems and I love to incorporate pieces of wisdom that I encounter into my own way of life.

On Facebook there was a video clip circulating of the Dali Lama speaking at the Glastonbury Festival's Pyramid Stage in Glastonbury, Somerset, UK on June 28, 2015. I am sure that you can find the clip if you search the Internet or YouTube. It is quite cute. He is about to turn 80 years old on July 6th. The group had organized for the Dali Lama to say a few words and blow out some candles on his birthday cake.

I have seen the Dali Lama speak in person at an event in Ottawa. His story is fascinating and worth learning about. When I was at that event many years ago, you could have heard a pin drop in the arena that held over 30,000 people. People just wanted to hear what this man had to say. There was no band. No music. Just a man and a sofa chair and his voice. Amazing evening.

He is full of laughter and joy and he makes me smile. While on stage addressing the fact that his birthday was coming up, he said, and I am paraphrasing, that the secret to true happiness is having concern for others. He says that his day is completely focused on the wellbeing of others. Imagine how this could change the world if we all stopped chasing material things to find happiness and looked toward each other instead.

If all of us were centrally focused on taking care of each other the world really would be a better place. Think of the way we walk through our day, rushing, cutting each other off in traffic. Walking through doors without looking behind us to see if we could hold it for the next person. Ignoring humanitarian issues all over the globe.

To live the way the Dali Lama lives would be too much for most of us, however we can try to be more mindful about the way in which we move through our space.

I guess I am lucky as I get to serve and teach my students every day, and being so centrally focused on their wellbeing has given me such happiness that it bubbles over into every-thing I do. I used to have a filing job in a company after I spent three hours teaching in the morning. I would arrive there every day full of joy and smiles only to be amazed by how down and depressed everyone else around me seemed to be feeling about their jobs. I actually had to downplay my joy in order to fit in. I hated that!

I see first hand how focusing on others brings true joy.

Try it. It may change your life.

Beth

# AT A SNAIL'S PACE

July 14, 2015

Last week I chose to leave the hustle and bustle of the building to eat my lunch outside on the grass and I happened to notice a snail nearby on the sidewalk. I can honestly say that I've never seen a live snail doing its thing. I've seen the abandoned shells and admired their colors but never before have I actually spent time watching them move. They truly are slow movers.

It appeared to me that this little guy was doing nothing, but as I studied him for 20 minutes, he had a clear mission in mind and it involved some vegetation. He was on his way to a piece of broken branch even though he appeared to be standing still. He was moving, very slowly. He was making real progress but you had to watch closely to see it.

My message today is about just that. At times, we are evolving so slowly that it appears we are not making any progress. In fitness, we want 'that body' right now and it's hard to wait for the results to manifest in our appearance. Some people give up on their training for this very reason. They expect to see perfection after a week in the gym but it really is about small, healthy changes over time. Fast, drastic weight loss that does not include lifelong changes to your eating patterns and exercise regime will result in the weight coming back on.

Losing weight is only one of the ways in which we measure success at the gym but it is the one that gets the most attention. There are other awesome changes that happen deep inside your body that are making you healthier. You cannot see them but every time you get yourself to the gym and lift some weights or do that yoga or aerobics class you are progressing. There are changes happening in your nervous system that optimize control of the muscles involved in exercise. This can be seen in your reflex responses. You are probably able to process information more quickly and get moving faster.

If you are strength training than your muscles are growing. Our muscles are not necessarily getting bigger but they become more defined. I am sure that my clients see huge changes in their ability to complete daily tasks. They tell me all of the time that their doctors are very impressed with their muscle strength, endurance and flexibility.

Your hearts are changing as well with regular exercise. The walls of the heart and ventricular cavity size can increase. Your resting blood pressure will improve. Your good cholesterol number will hopefully increase and the bad number will hopefully go down. Your bone density will improve with regular strength training, which is so important for all of us as we age. We cannot see these physiological adaptations to our bodies but like our friend the snail, we are progressing on our road to better health, slowly.

Slow and steady wins the race every single time.

Beth

# ARE YOU BREATHING?

June 18, 2015

Are you breathing?

I ask my students this several times during our workouts together. It is amazing to me how many people forget to breathe while training. My mission is to get them to release built up tension and help them to get through the class safely and effectively. What I do notice is that many people struggle to take in a deep breath. Often their in-breath is very shallow. I watch as they must scrunch up their shoulders in order to fill their lungs even just a bit.

Try this:

Sit tall on the edge of your chair and breathe in deeply through your nose. First, your nose may be blocked so you need to try to clear that in order to breathe properly. Try to breathe in for a count of four and then exhale through your mouth for the same count but this time pretend you are breathing out through a straw and control the flow of the breath. When we practice this, we can actually improve our ability to take in more oxygen and as a result we will have more energy and feel calmer.

In class, I ask students to check in with their breath as it is an indication of how we are doing physically. If our breath is short and choppy, we may be pushing ourselves too hard. As a way to remember to breathe I tell my students to exhale with the hard part of any exercise. For example, in a push up, do the exhale when you are pushing away from the floor or surface.

Try the following exercise before you get out of bed before the mind starts to take over and you begin to worry about the day ahead. I want you to place one hand on your heart and one hand on your abdomen. Slowly inhale, feeling your belly rise, ribs rise and chest rise and then reverse this by exhaling until there is no more air left in your lungs. I want you to do this while counting to four with the in breath and down from four with the out breath. Just focus on the quality of your breath. Eventually you will be able to increase the length of your in breath. I know this to be true because when I first started doing this exercise four years ago, my breath was very shallow. It felt like my chest was going to burst if I tried to take in any more air.

Clients have reported to me that simply doing this every morning has helped them to lower their blood pressure and improve their quality of life. Isn't that what we all want?

Check in with your breath several times today. You will be happy you did!

Beth

# BELIEVE IN YOURSELF

October 14, 2015

Personal Training is a balance of tough love and compassion. People come to me to make changes to their physical bodies but what often ends up happening is a transformation of the mind.

"If you tell yourself that you can't, you won't!" I find myself saying this quite often in my group classes as well as in my private sessions. Attitude really is everything. It is my job to give clients the tools and knowledge to execute the exercise but if they have already decided that they are going to fail, they will.

Ask yourself if you are actually sabotaging your own efforts to change your circumstances. I see this in all areas of my teaching. Sometimes when faced with a new challenge we revert back to the 'stories' that we tell ourselves. "Oh I cannot do that. I have never been able to do that exercise. I cannot change."

Yesterday we were working on balance challenges as we prepare for slippery winter conditions. I want to make sure that my clients are steady on their feet and part of the way that I do this is to put them in a safe situation that demands the recruitment of their stabilizing muscles. Once I cue how to stay steady, most of the class will execute the moves perfectly. I can then see the students who are laughing or growing increasingly frustrated as they fall back into their old patterns of thought. I can literally see their thoughts on their faces. Their whole appearance changes. They are exhibiting signs of self doubt.

So how do we break these self sabotaging thought patterns? Whenever I want to make a change, I create little rhymes or mantras that I repeat to myself. No one has to know you are doing this but it will help to snap you out of your pattern. One that I commonly use is 'life is good, life is easy, all good things are coming to me.' I recommend that you make your own. I have written about five mantras up to this point. I started in 2010 when my life was most challenging. It pulled me through those tough times and now I create new ones whenever I feel the need to prop myself up.

You will change your life by changing your thoughts.

Beth

# NEVER ASSUME

November 21, 2018

Last night's heavy snowfall made the commute to work quite stressful today. As I was driving to work I couldn't help but grumble about all of the people slowing things down because of bad habits. When we don't clear off the tops of our cars, it's hazardous to the people behind. All drivers know this and yet many just jump in and go, but have you ever wondered why people don't clean off the car completely? I have always just assumed laziness was the reason or tardiness and I believe that this is true in the majority of cases, but yesterday I had my eyes opened by a lady who I meet quite frequently at the gym. She is in her mid fifties and is in a wheelchair but she rarely never misses her workout despite bad weather!

I had to tell her how impressed I was at her determination. "Oh," she said, "it's hard on days like today, I'm not going to lie. The worst part is I feel badly because I cannot clean off the roof of my van and people drive by giving me dirty looks and cursing." Her words stopped me in my tracks. We rarely know what someone else is struggling with in this life. We can debate and criticize the behavior all we want but perhaps we need to know all of the facts before we make any judgement. Yes, it is annoying to drive behind a snow-covered car but after speaking with my friend from the locker room, I'm not going to be so quick to be rude to the drivers around me anymore.

Have a great day and while you are at it make someone smile with a kind word. It goes a long way...maybe even offer to help someone you know who might need a hand this winter.

Beth

# BE CAREFUL ABOUT JUDGEMENT

October 5, 2016

I'm different. Perhaps because I've been small all of my life and considered to be weak due to my size, I know better than to judge anyone based on their body shape or age for that matter.

As a line dance instructor I often go to YouTube to find new material to share with my clients. This week I found two videos of men dancing and I was immediately impressed. I only have a few men in my dance classes so it encouraged me to see this and I started dancing right along with the video! I then found the steps for the dances and prepared to teach them to my students. I also sent the videos along to my students for them to enjoy.

More than one of the students came back with comments about the size of the dancers and it completely shocked me. The comments were not mean but just the fact that they brought up their size, instead of how great they were moving, disappointed me. I also get this from students in their 50s who hear that I train people in their late 70s and early 80s. Before they even give the class a try, they have decided that they do not want to be with 'old' people. Again, I am shocked.

I do my best to motivate people of all sizes and ages to get moving and exercising. Their strength, determination and talent continue to inspire me on a daily basis.

Beth

# LAUGHTER IN YOGA

November 3, 2015

It happens. People can start to laugh unexpectedly in yoga class where traditionally the tone of the class is introspective, quiet and meditative. This occurred in both of my yoga classes yesterday and for some people it provides a much needed stress release. It can be disruptive to others though so we have to make sure it does not get out of hand.

The poses can be challenging and some of them look quite silly. When I am introducing a new pose, I know that there are going to be people who are ready for the challenge and those who are not interested at all. As the teacher, I can see that there are at least three different levels of capability in my class and the important thing for me is to keep offering opportunities for growth, to those who want a bit more out of their class experience.

Everyone has arrived in my class for a different reason. Some students have been told by their doctor that they have to relieve stress and become more flexible. They are often injured and so I have to make sure that they know not to push themselves to the point of discomfort, and to always come out of the pose should they feel badly. Some students want to see all that yoga has to offer them and they are fit and ready to try new poses. For this type of client, they need to see that the class is progressing over the 12-week session.

The challenge for me is to keep the non-injured, perfectly fit individual in great shape so that they do not become injured. The focus cannot always be on the 'beginner' or the injured student because I have to keep the more fit students interested and progressing. My mission is to make sure that everyone feels safe and that everyone has options!

Make sure that whatever category you fall into, that you do not impose your situation on the rest of the class by making comments about the pose being 'stupid' or 'too hard' or 'impossible.' While it is okay to laugh quietly and smile and revert into a pose that feels safe for you, please encourage others who are willing to step out of their comfort zone and grow. We are in a learning environment after all. This is the place to try new things, laugh and grow.

Beth

# TOO HAPPY?

May 26, 2015

Some people find me to be sickeningly happy. I am not everyone's cup of tea. In fact, the one and only complaint I have ever received on an evaluation form said that I am too demonstrative about my happiness. "She is too happy!"

I took that to heart and the next time I taught that class I tried to be more reserved. I did not smile. I tried to be serious. At the end of the class, once everyone had left, I told myself that if this is what the students want, then I have to quit. Well, luckily I simply gave up that class at the end of the session and did not give up my career.

My life is not all butterflies and roses. It has been wonderful so far but I have struggled as well. When I was going through a rough patch a few years ago, after the death of my parents and some job dissatisfaction, my health started to wane. It seemed as though nothing was going right. I found myself sinking into a hole of misery. I found myself at the book store in search of some words of wisdom and Pema Chodron's book caught my eye, *The Places ThatScare You – A Guide to Fearlessness in Difficult Times.*

What I learned from Pema's words is that what we focus on expands, so if we are feeling miserable and we focus on it, we will begin to only see misery which will make us feel worse and so on. The cycle is vicious and it leads to poor health in body and mind. Well I had seen enough misery so I chose to do whatever it took to turn my life around.

I chose to focus on the things that were going right in my life even if they were small. In time, I began to see more and more amazing things, even though I was still feeling crappy a lot of the time. My day was filled with half misery and half joy which was better than all misery. I chose to be positive. I chose to be happy. It was hard work to pull myself out of the despair but I knew that I still wanted to make some of my dreams come true, so I had to make a change. Please note that I realize I am one of the lucky ones as not everyone can climb out of depression so easily. Always seek medical assistance whenever you feel you need more help.

Now my life is filled with such joy that I really have a hard time not smiling constantly. I do not want to look like a complete idiot but I have learned to find joy in tiny things, like a hot cup of coffee or tea uninterrupted. A good read on a rainy day. Glorious sunsets and sunrises. Smiles from friends, family and strangers.

You see, life can be so disappointing if we let it. You can pile up all the crap going wrong in your life and find many people who will help you to do this! "Misery loves company" is not just a saying, it is true because it is easy to add up life's challenges. Do you catch yourself saying any of the following statement? "I do not have enough money. My kids don't listen. This job sucks. I am so fat. I hate my life." It can be very hard to stop telling ourselves those things and find any instance of joy when we are so consumed by unhappiness.

With baby steps anyone can turn their life around. I started by changing my focus, searching for positivity. I began my day trying to come up with just one thing that I was happy for, even if it was just 'my comfortable bed.' Each day I would try to add one more item and then when I heard myself slipping into complaining mode I would say to myself, "But wait, I have a beautiful home and a lovely family and that is all that matters right now, I can keep going."

It gets easier and easier, especially with wonderful books like Pema's. I am not a Buddhist, but I love reading how different traditions handle life and then I choose to incorporate into my life, what works for me! If you are a bit down and need to try something new, pick up her book.

I hope this helps.

Beth

# A MESSAGE FOR THE LADIES

August 6, 2015

I cannot speak to what it is to be a man in this world but I can say that as a woman, I personally have been very judgemental about my appearance, and my teaching experience tells me that I am not alone.

A cartoon was given to me by one of my students who has a great sense of humour. It depicts a slim woman looking in the mirror who sees herself as quite large (fat) and then beside it there is a depiction of a large man looking in the mirror and he sees himself as fit with six pack abs. Women typically have body image issues whereas many of the men that I meet in my work are not as critical of their midriff bulges.

Realistically, you need to know that men store their fat viscerally, that is around their organs, while women store their fat subcutaneously, just under their skin. So I have had male clients smack their big bellies and tell me that they have rock hard abs despite their size and therefore they are in great shape and don't need my personal training services.

What this cartoon tells me is that men can exhibit a wonderful sense of self confidence that I sometimes wish I had myself. No matter what their shape or size, some men can look in the mirror and see a strong, fit individual looking back at them and be happy with that! While the man's perception of himself in this cartoon is delusional, I see so many women struggling with a low sense of self that I wish women could feel a bit better about their bodies.

Do not get me wrong. The man in this cartoon is at serious risk for developing many potentially life threatening health problems. The struggle that I face in my work, is that men like him feel so well that it is hard to convince them that they need to get into the gym and shed the weight, while I have many female students who are fit but pushing themselves to be thinner!

Becoming fit is not just a matter of working with our physical bodies, it is also a bit of a mind game. My job is to help my students to feel good when they are in my classes so that they continue to work toward achieving optimal health. Please note however that we have to take care of our thoughts about ourselves, just as much as we need to work out our bodies.

Ask yourself what is driving you to work out?

Remember that becoming healthy is not just about getting thin, it is about feeling good in body, mind and soul. Work on all three and you will feel fabulous.

Beth

# GREAT ADVICE ON LIVING WELL

May 20, 2016

I just listened to a TED Talk that was given by Anita Moorjani, a woman who died and came back to life. What interested me about this talk was the advice she shared on how to live our lives. I realize that many of you may not believe that there is life after death, however I feel that her advice is valuable and worth sharing. Anita tells us that we need to focus on five important things while we are living.

- We need to focus on loving ourselves. It is true that we spend more time criticizing ourselves than we spend forgiving our mistakes and accepting ourselves as we are.

- She tells us to live our lives fearlessly. We often think that fear is protecting us but she claims it is fear that holds us back from living a full and happy life.

- "The most important spiritual activity," in Anita's words, is finding our joy. We are born smiling and laughing but some of us stop doing this spontaneously. She wants us to seek out joy for we are meant to be happy and laughing while we are here.

- Life is a gift and we need to look at all the challenges that come our way as a way to learn the value of our lives. My modest health concerns used to drag me down but I do see them as a gift now. They taught me to live each day as if it is a gift.

- Anita says that it is important that we always be ourselves and embrace our uniqueness. This will ultimately lead us to find joy.

Beth

# YOUR LIFE IN SIX WORDS!

May 31, 2016

The idea is not mine but I find the challenge interesting. We all have stories to tell but can you simplify your story into six little words? Here are some examples that I found from an old Oprah magazine that are quite creative. (The Oprah Magazine, February 2012, volume 13. Number 2. pp. 126-127)

*"Every 20 years, I reinvent myself."* – Wahana Vellutini.
*"Abandoned at 5. Learning to thrive."* – Melinda Hui.
*"I am more than a twin."*- Diane Campbell
*"Surfing life's ripples, wishing for waves."* – Karen Barbier
*"Might as well eat that cookie."* – Paula Deen
*"I have time to fix this."* – Taneika Head

The beauty of this exercise is that it gets you to think about your life, where you have been and how far you have come. We only have a few minutes to make an impression when we meet someone for the first time. At the gym, I can predict the degree of success that someone will have in my class based on our initial meeting. How do you feel about yourself? What are your goals? What can you tell me about yourself that will highlight your strengths and weaknesses?

When you are speaking, I' m looking at the words that you use to describe yourself. They tell me where you are on your fitness journey and how easy or hard it may be to help you achieve your goals.

In my work as a fitness instructor, clients often have very little time to convey their thoughts to me as classes empty out and others arrive. People often run up to me to get their point across. I do my best to tune in and be present for everyone at that point. I must admit that I really appreciate the kind words that come my way on a daily basis. I know that those people have given great thought and chosen their words carefully.

I do my best to forget the words that are meant to cause pain. Those moments are difficult as I have to shake off the feeling and turn around within three minutes and use my words to encourage, support and inspire.

Condensing my words is a way of life for me. Working with the public, I must be careful. I cannot always speak my mind and maybe that is a good thing.

Perhaps more of us need to hold in some of our ideas, process them properly and fully consider their impact before releasing them into the universe.

Try this exercise. Share it with me privately. It may give me a bit more insight into who you are at this moment.

My life in six words: "Dance. Eat. Laugh. Repeat with love." – Beth Oldfield

Beth

# LIFE IS A GOOD TEACHER

November 18, 2015

"Life is a good teacher and a good friend."

These are the wise words of Pema Chodron from her book, *When Things Fall Apart. Heart Advice for Difficult Times.*

We have a tendency to want things to stay the same. Especially when things are going well. What Pema teaches us in her book is that life is always changing, always in transition. Sadness comes when we expect that we can control events and have to learn time and time again, that this is not possible. The trick Pema says is in not hardening into resentment or bitterness. We have to catch ourselves before we go down that path as it will lead to more suffering and sadness.

I am facing a new challenge but what I noticed over the last 48 hours is that I am appreciating the little things more. I see that I had come to take things for granted and I needed a bit of a wake up call. I pride myself on living in the moment but even one who is so tuned in can get lured into thinking that life is always going to be humming along perfectly! Today I was thankful for things that I had forgotten to be thankful for. I learned a great lesson over the last few days.

Take nothing for granted. Walk a bit slower. Share time with those you love. Sit a bit longer. Take in the sun and the warmth and be thankful for every minute that is your own.

Beth

# GOOD NEWS STORIES

June 13, 2018

My students regularly share their personal stories with me and I'm most inspired when someone tells me how exercise has improved their life. I can see firsthand how strong and flexible my students are in class but I love hearing how the movements that we practice so often affect their daily activities. Many people tell me how regular exercise improves their sport performance but I also hear plenty of 'near miss' stories or stories where disaster was avoided.

Last week, one of my students avoided serious injury and she believes that exercise class was the reason! She was returning home from a workout at the gym when she slipped on a freshly stained deck surface. There was no sign or rope to mark off the area and so she proceeded to walk across it normally but quickly found herself off balance. She was very happy to tell me that her legs were strong enough to keep her from doing the splits and I would add that all of the balance work that we have been doing in class over the last year added to her stability.

Injuries happen when rarely used muscles are called upon to work quickly, under load. Because we have been strengthening her inner thighs, knees, hips and core muscles her body was ready to catch her and keep her safe. This news makes me very happy!

A few days ago, another of my students caught his toe on the edge of something as he was exiting class but he was able to quickly get his leg out in front to catch himself before hitting the ground. I know that in his case all of the stretching that we have been doing to keep his hips flexible allowed him to move with fluidity to avoid injury.

And still another one of my students was rushing down her driveway to get to the car two weeks ago when her foot sank down into a hole causing her to trip. Her ankle was sprained but not broken and she believes that all of the foot strengthening that we have been doing saved her from spending the summer in a cast. She also recovered very quickly and was back in class one week later!

If you ever find yourself questioning whether or not you need to formally exercise, please know that taking care of yourself and all of your muscles is incredibly valuable in more ways than one. Get to class!

I love hearing these stories. Keep them coming.

Beth

# PEGGY'S ESSENTRICS® SUCCESS STORY!

January 15, 2020

One of my newest students just wrote me a lovely email describing the success that she has enjoyed after taking my Essentrics® class for 12 weeks. These stories encourage me to continue teaching this amazing program! Peggy has suffered with pain in her lower back, neck and shoulders for many years. Her work requires that she stand for long periods of time and she has been seeing her chiropractor every three to four weeks for adjustments over the last 26 years. These treatments, coupled with regular exercise that included Yoga, Pilates and dance has helped Peggy to keep the pain to a minimum.

Peggy joined my new Essentrics® class in Rigaud, Quebec last September and after participating two times a week for an hour each time, she arrived at one of the last classes of the session with a huge smile on her face. "My chiropractor said I need to thank you Beth, because for the first time ever, my back is in perfect alignment! I believe that stretching is the magic solution for my back issues." I was so happy for her and so pleased that the Essentrics® techniques were able to complete the healing process.

In our classes we move every single joint the way it was intended to move, and as such we lubricate and revitalize parts of our body that otherwise get stiff because of lifestyle choices and inactivity. The workouts are gentle in the sense that you work at your own intensity level, but do not interpret this to mean that the exercise is easy or somehow ineffective. I have been teaching Essentrics® now for over two years and I have seen amazing results in my own flexibility, and a reduction in pain in my back, shoulders and feet. Life is too short to spend any of it in pain. Maybe I can help!

Beth

# A STROKE WON'T STOP JOE!

March 16, 2018

In April of last year, I wrote a blog about a neighbour and friend of mine named Joe, entitled "Exercise as Insurance." I wrote it after learning that Joe (mid-sixties) had suffered a severe stroke. I had spoken to him about ten years beforehand, saying that I was worried about the stress level in his life and how it might be affecting his health. I wanted him to start training with me in my home studio classes. Joe was at the top of his field, working long hours in a fast paced profession that demanded excellence. He was always running and travelling long distances for work and felt that he had no time to focus on himself.

Does that sound familiar to you? Maybe you know someone in your life who fits this profile or maybe it is you yourself who makes everything else a priority instead of taking the time to eat well, exercise and get adequate rest.

Joe suffered a stroke on March 7th, 2017. At the time he was completely paralyzed down one side of his body and he was told that he would never walk again. He had to eat through a tube inserted in his stomach and he could not breathe on his own. The doctors stood over him and said, "There is nothing we can do. You will be like this for the rest of your life." I get choked up whenever I think about this because he has proven them all wrong.

By May he was walking around our neighbourhood with a cane that he called his friend, Bob. By July he was asking if he could train in my basement. I was reluctant at first but remarkably he was able to get down the stairs and lift some lite weights. Getting onto the floor to do some simple exercises was quite a workout in itself, not to mention getting back up again. I loaned him some weights and gave him some guidance and he continued on his own in his home. By September he was walking without Bob and in late October he joined my class with my five other students.

I was very nervous about how he would keep up but there is one thing I have learned about Joe. Don't tell him he cannot do something because he is stubborn and he will try until he gets it. So I learned to tell him if I thought something was too dangerous for him and he learned to listen when the tone of my voice was stern. Otherwise, he basically did our workout with very little adaptation. He would do fewer repetitions of weights and sit and take breaks when his legs grew tired but he would always get back up and finish.

In December, I introduced Essentrics® to my home studio class and that is when Joe really began to shine, as he was able to do most of the movements right along with the rest of the class. There was very little need to give him alternative exercises. He simply stopped when he grew tired and got back up when he felt he rested.

Today, he squealed in delight during one of the calf stretches, where our feet are staggered quite far apart, with one foot in front and the other in back. This stance can be quite challenging for stroke patients when one leg is weaker especially because we are tipped forward at  he hip, one arm reaching forward, the other extending backward. I place a chair near Joe which he usually uses for balance but today he was doing it on his own. I was focused on the other students (simply because he wants it that way) when Joe yelled out "Hey, look at my balance Beth!" He was standing on his own, with no hands on the chair, reaching forward and backward.

Joe has continued to surprise and impress me with his progress and it is directly attributed to his positive attitude. No one is going to tell him he cannot do something. He believes he can get back to his old self! The medical professionals examined him on the anniversary of his stroke and the top specialist in Montreal said that Joe's story is one in a million. He should have been dead by now. He is completely shocked that Joe proved all of the doctors wrong. Which by the way was Joe's personal mission. Early last Spring I would run out to greet him whenever I caught him walking by on the street and he would say through tears, "I'm gonna prove those "bleeping" doctors wrong!"

Congratulations Joe!

Believe and you will achieve.

Beth

# PART SIX

# GOAL ACCOMPLISHMENT

I am a forward thinker with my eyes clearly set on the next milestone even before I have completed the challenge at hand. Some people find this difficult to understand as I always seem to be working towards something, never sitting still for long. The truth is I have this nagging feeling that there is so much to get done with little time to waste. Perhaps because I was raised by older parents who lived their later years in poor health, I fear that my able-bodied time might be predetermined by my genes, so I'm rushing to achieve as many of my goals as possible with the valuable time that I have been given.

You might not believe this but I wake up each morning genuinely excited because I know that the first hour of my day I will be working on one of my many projects. I make my coffee and head up to my creative space and without fail, I log in a certain amount of time each day making my dreams a reality. There is no secret formula to goal achievement that will work for everyone, but I do know that it requires consistent effort over time. Maybe you can get up earlier or change your nighttime routine to fit in some time for working toward your goals.

The students who have achieved their fitness goals in my classes are the ones who never make excuses and show up without fail. I wish there was a way around it but it is the cold hard truth. No one is going to do the work for you so I hope that this section of my book will provide some of the motivation and inspiration that you might need to keep moving toward a healthier life.

# WRITE DOWN YOUR REASON WHY

May 23, 2018

There are many reasons why people head to the gym or hire personal trainers. I find the reasons fascinating. Everyone has a different 'why' and it is important for each of us to remember our own reason because it is what pulls us through on difficult days.

As we know, it is easy to find excuses to skip a workout. Truth be told not everyone finds exercise as enjoyable as I do. I love working out but most people don't and it can be a slippery slope when we make that first excuse. It then gets easier and easier to find excuses so I encourage people to write down their reasons for exercising and put it up where you can see it regularly.

Maybe you are trying to get healthier for your kids so you can be a better part of their lives. Put up a picture of your kids and write your reason underneath.

Maybe you are trying to lose weight so that you can look fabulous at the upcoming wedding or reunion. Write down your reason on a copy of the invitation.

Maybe you simply want to fit into that awesome pair of jeans you bought two years ago. Hang them front and center with a note stating the date that you want to wear them comfortably.

Maybe your buddy (60 years old) suffered a heart attack playing hockey and you want to avoid such a crisis. Hang his picture and write an affirmation to him that you will keep exercising in his honor.

Maybe you have to keep moving to keep your arthritis from crippling your life or your diabetes levels constant. Maybe your doctor told that you are morbidly obese and are at risk for an early death. Maybe you are on a mission to prove your doctors wrong when they told you that you would never walk again!

Every single one of those 'whys' has been expressed to me in the last year. They are all different but all incredibly good reasons to get moving on a daily basis.

Hang your 'why' up where you can see it and hopefully it will help to motivate you on those days when you feel like skipping your workout.

Beth

# IT'S ALL ABOUT CONSISTENCY!

October 5, 2020

When it comes to goal accomplishment, consistent effort is required.

As I was teaching Essentrics® last Friday, it occurred to me that I was able to lift my leg higher during the kick sequence than I had been able to do previously. This means that all of the dedicated work that I have been putting in is finally starting to pay off. Sometimes in fitness we think that we have to make drastic changes to our lives in order to achieve our goals, but in truth the small, consistent, daily efforts are what bring about big, physical changes in our body.

COVID-19 knocked many of us off track in March but I can see remarkable progress in the health of my students who have kept up their fitness routines virtually from the safety of their homes. Is it perfect? No. But there is never going to be a *perfect* time to work on your goals or your projects. You just have to commit to a small amount of time each day and you will succeed.

Yesterday, I decided to get back to a few of my projects that were put aside in the Spring. You see I had fallen into the trap of thinking that it had to be all or nothing. That unless I could devote hours a day toward my goal, there was no point. Well Friday opened my eyes. It is the little bits of time that we spend on our projects that move us toward completion. You do not need to move mountains, you just need to take some steps every single day toward reaching the top.

One of my projects is to take my grandmother's cookbook and turn it into a hard cover book for the family. There are 96 recipes in her notebook, all out of order of course, so this is a big task. As the writer in the family, I believe that part of my reason for being is to record the stories of my ancestors. This is just one of the many projects on my To Do list, and instead of feeling weighed down by the magnitude of the final product, I will instead focus twenty minutes a day on getting the work done, and I will celebrate these efforts along the way.

What can you begin to work on today?

Beth

# ACHIEVE YOUR GOAL IN FIVE EASY STEPS

April 24, 2019

Whether you want to lose ten pounds, publish a book, build your dream home or take that long awaited trip to somewhere exotic, it all starts with naming the goal and setting your sights on completion!

Often we have many things that we want to accomplish but we keep them to ourselves. This past week, I learned about another friend who has just been diagnosed with stage 4 cancer, so what is on my mind today is just how short life can be and how we have to get busy if we want to live our best lives! And for me, living my best life is making my dreams come true!

I have managed to accomplish quite a bit in the last few years and people often express their amazement at my achievements so I thought I would share my strategies.

1.  Make a list of things that you want to accomplish. Dream big. Some people refer to this as making a 'bucket list.'

2.  Then find images from magazines that represent your goals and stick them to a big poster board, naming each one in big letters. For example: 'Publish a book of short stories' beside an image of a stack of books. Put this board where you will see it daily. This will keep you focused on your goals.

3.  From your list or vision board, pick one to three things that you think you could accomplish this week and build time into your schedule to make it happen. Starting with the easiest goals is motivating because success is the best motivator!

4. At the end of this week, pick a few more easily achievable goals but also one thing that you could accomplish within the next month or two and one thing that you could do within one year.

5. MAKE time to get it done. I personally alter my work schedule because I can. I get up earlier to study or exercise. I socialize a bit less and turn down invitations to just 'chill' with friends. I don't have a television which leaves me plenty of time to be productive. Slow and steady wins the race each and every time. So don't think that spending half an hour to an hour working on your goals is unproductive. A book is written one page at a time.

I hope this helps!

Beth

# NEW YEAR'S RESOLUTION HELP

January 2, 2019

If you're like me you have made your resolutions and have come up with some goals for 2019. Personally, I woke up in a panic today, wondering how I am going to achieve all that I have planned! Aside from needing to rest more, which is the flip side to being a busy fitness instructor, I want to complete my novel, work on my memoir and tell the fascinating story of my grandmother's journey to Canada! I want to create more videos and another fitness book.

One of the best ways that I have found to deal with goals is quite old school. Map out your daily activities, listing the things that you have to do and the time of day when they need to get done, and see where you can fit in 20 to 30 minutes of time for yourself. Then take a piece of cardboard, listing the days of the week and plan what you will work on each day during that 20-30 minute time slot. Put this 'activities map' where you can see it all of the time and it should keep you on track.

This tactic has helped me to complete many projects over the years. The trick is it has to be visible. This tactic is quite helpful when you have many projects to work on but it can be used for exercise as well. I have always told you that variety is the key to good health. You can plan out your activity and this helps some people to stay on track.

I have the most energy in the morning, so I get up earlier to work on my dreams. If you are perked up later in the day then choose that as your 'get things done' time. No matter what your goal might be, there is always a few minutes within the day where you can do a small bit toward achieving the goal. When it comes to fitness goals, slow and steady wins the race each and every time. Don't make huge weight loss goals and expect to achieve it in one month but instead, promise to work out in some way each day, without fail. Clients who refuse to let anything get in the way of their exercise date with themselves see the best results.

Beth

# ARE YOUR EXPECTATIONS REALISTIC?

November 10, 2016

When you start a new fitness regime, I want you to consider your expectations.

I generally see three types of clients:

1. People who haven't worked out in a long time and want to lose weight and be 'toned' by the weekend or in two weeks.

2. People who want to get fit but aren't willing to break a sweat or push themselves in order to do so.

3. People who see the need to get in shape and are completely committed to doing all that they can to improve their health.

Students in the third category are the ones who succeed and keep returning to the gym. I'm happy to say that my classes are filled with these types of clients, however I meet people from the first two categories every few months. Generally, their expectations are unrealistic and there is very little that I can do to help them to succeed.

I recently worked very hard to make a newcomer feel welcome during their first class and I was saddened to learn that she will not be returning.

People decide to quit for many reasons. Sometimes it is because they are intimidated by the abilities of the students around them. Perhaps they feel that they will never be as good as everyone else so why bother? Or maybe they didn't like the feeling of stepping out of their comfort zone. It can be hard to be the new person in the room. Exercise can also bring on some muscular pain. Many people cannot tolerate the initial stiffness and discomfort that is normal when you take up a new activity. Maybe the client did not appreciate the music or the movements.

It is for these reasons that I urge all new students to give each class at least three attempts before giving up. I change my music every class so chances are that you will hear something that you like the next time you visit. I also vary the exercises and if you attend regularly you will feel like you are improving. If the teacher was not your 'cup of tea,' I still encourage you to try again because he/she may have been having a bad day. It happens to all of us and we all deserve a second chance. Take the time to address any of these concerns with the teacher.

If you are just starting out, commit to exercising at least three times per week, for three months. Hire a personal trainer to assist you in achieving your goals or speak to your group fitness instructor for advice. Remember that our mission is your success. That is why we are there!

Beth

# MAKE YOUR PLANS NOW

December 4, 2019

I encourage my students to commit to a program that will keep them active before the weather turns cold and icy because if you make plans now, you are more likely to keep moving and stay healthy. Many of my students travel to the south to escape the harsh winters that we experience in Quebec, Canada. The older I get the more I start to understand the appeal of this yearly migration. There seems to be more ice and less snow than in years past and this makes getting around challenging. The concern I have is that if people do not make plans for their fitness from January to April, they will fall out of their fitness routine. Why does this matter? Couldn't we all take three or four months off from working out?

In my experience, watching from the front of the class for the last twenty years, those students who plan ahead and quite frankly, never miss their workout unless they are ill, are the ones who are in the best physical and mental shape. Even if they catch a cold, they are better able to fight it off because they are in good physical condition. While I believe that it is healthy and necessary at times to take vacations and only work out sporadically during that time, completely stopping your exercise regime for months at a time sets your progress back to zero and getting back from that point is hard work, so hard in fact that many people never go back.

If you are travelling, you can purchase my fitness videos so that you can continue to work out while away or do some research to find out about the local gyms and their fitness class options that are available near your destination. Either way, please stay active.

Beth

# "FAKE IT UNTIL YOU MAKE IT"

September 22, 2015

As many of you know, I have started a new job teaching English to adult students, who need are trying to obtain their high school diploma. The students I am working with are for the most part wonderful kids who just need a second chance to move on with their lives.

Last week, they all did oral presentations in front of the class and yesterday I gave them their grades. The class average was 80% but there were a few who barely passed. In speaking with these kids in particular, I told them that their body language during the presentation was giving off a vibe that they were shy or afraid and that the reading of their cue cards with heads down, made them impossible to hear.

I know that some of the kids were terrified to be at the front of the class. As I spend 20+ hours a week speaking to crowds, I know how stressful this can be but part of being successful is believing in yourself! I told them to "fake it until they make it."

I had to explain this statement to mean that at times in life our coach or our boss may ask us if we can do something for the team. We may be worried about the outcome but our leader does not want to hear that we cannot do it. If we act worried, he/she may question why we were selected for the job and regret this decision! We have to try and try our best. We have to believe that we can do something and walk with an air of confidence. This is half the battle. In time, the rest will come with hard work!

When my fitness students are learning a new aerobic routine or dance, we have to stumble through the steps and practice to get the movements just right. During the weekly classes, we must believe that we can achieve our goals before we even try.

If you tell yourself you 'cannot' do something, you will not do it for sure. The choice is up to you.

See you soon where we will be faking the moves together until we get them just right!

Have a great day,

Beth

# EXERCISE IS UNCOMFORTABLE

November 11, 2016

I am very clear with all of my students that they are the boss when it comes to whether or not to perform certain exercises. "If something feels wrong or painful, do not do it." When I say this in my group fitness classes, it is a way for me to make sure that people understand how to be aware of their own limits. People come to group classes for many different reasons. Some are there just to socialize, while others have serious fitness goals. For this reason, I make sure that my students learn to listen to their own bodies.

Exercise is meant to make you uncomfortable to a certain degree. If you are there to try to lose weight or become more flexible, you will need to step out of your comfort zone to achieve your goal. You may need to increase your heart rate to burn more calories or you may need assistance in reaching a bit further in stretch classes. Ultimately though, no one should push you beyond what you deem to be your acceptable limit. We all have to decide how far to push ourselves. The good thing about group classes is that they give you an idea of what others are doing to step out of their comfort zone. Working with a personal trainer can help you establish what you need to do to meet your targets, based on your specific situation. Just be aware that your current state of health is largely a result of you being comfortable to some degree.

To make positive changes to your current situation, you will need to spend time feeling uncomfortable. Soon you will establish a new normal for yourself. A new zone of healthier living and joy!

Beth

# OCTOBER-FITTEST MONTH OF THE YEAR?

October 12, 2016

"October is the fittest month of the year." I heard this statement on CTV News from Ottawa last night.

At first the statement seemed a bit ridiculous but as I considered what they were saying it made sense. If people join the gym in September and actually stick with it for six to eight weeks, I would agree that they could be in better shape than when they first walked in.

The report went on to explain that the upcoming holiday season, coupled with parties and drinking and eating, results in weight gain from now until Christmas. During the winter months many people hibernate in their homes because of poor weather and dangerous driving conditions and the gyms are generally not as busy in the Spring because people are working in their gardens.

The news story suggested that because we feel so good in October, we should make our New Year's Resolutions now!

Perhaps we should make a commitment to keep coming to classes no matter what the weather brings, maybe we should vow to eat less and move more during the holiday season? Maybe our resolutions would have nothing to do with weight at all.

What would you do today to make your life even better? Give it a try.

Beth

# HOW COMMITTED ARE YOU?

May 2, 2018

I ask this as a serious question because personal trainers are judged constantly by the success of their clients, but your success (should you be looking to get fit) is directly related to how committed you are to the process of getting into better physical shape.

For example, how would you go about hiring a trainer? After ensuring that the trainer in question holds up-to-date credentials, you would then want to pick someone who comes highly recommended. Maybe this trainer helped a friend of yours to shed unwanted weight. Trainers are judged by the quality of the product that we put out. However, it works both ways. Trainers need to be choosy about who they select to train because in the end, we are only hired if we have been successful.

Years ago, I slowed down my personal training business in favor of small group personal training because I was lousy at choosing clients. I was too eager to help everyone and I quickly learned that there are two types of people. Those who are willing to put in the hard, challenging work no matter how they feel on any given day, and those who want to say that they are working with a trainer, but really they cancel more than they sweat.

Commitment is the most important part of fitness training which means that even when you don't feel like it, you must tie on those shoes and get to the session. Trainers are committing their time to you and you must commit in equal measure. Yes, I understand that life gets in the way but what I know for sure is that when you begin to miss training sessions for less than important reasons, you are setting yourself up for failure.

As I said, I rarely do one-on-one sessions now because I grew tired of cancellations for lame reasons. That is the honest truth. The small group environment has a built in mechanism called 'accountability'. When someone misses class, I don't need to say a thing. The other members of the group do all the talking and supporting for me. "Where were you?" "We missed you?" "Hey, see you next week right?"

Some clients prefer to train when there a few people in the group because they can see each other's progress and this motivates them to continue. It can also be motivating to be around your peers and measure yourself up. "Oh wow, I need to up my game" or "Okay, I am not doing too badly. I can keep going!"

I am so lucky that the small groups that I started years ago still continue today. The members are very supportive, kind and completely committed to the process of getting into shape. No excuses! And we laugh so much that working out is fun. Really fun! Find what works for you and commit today!

Beth

# FRIENDS WILL HOLD YOU ACCOUNTABLE!

November 17, 2016

Though I love to work out, I have to accept that many people don't. So what can you do if you hate breaking a sweat but know that you have to exercise to stay healthy? The answer is simple: find a workout buddy. My most successful students are the ones who come to the gym with their friends or meet them there. There are a few students who travel in a pack at my gym and attend the classes that their friends are attending, because right after the workout they socialize over coffee. Their commitment to each other is what gets them to the gym time and time again.

When we go it alone, it can be hard to justify leaving our families or spouses but if we have a 'date' to meet a friend at the gym, it is somehow easier to convince those around us to let us go. We are also less likely to disappoint a friend by not showing up. I am amazed how much my students care for one another and how much they worry when someone is missing. In my opinion, it is these friendships that guarantee our success at the gym. Even if you do not have someone to go to the gym with right now, attend classes and reach out to people. Introduce yourself and open yourself up to change.

We simply need to get moving and as far as I am concerned the rest will fall into place. Going through the motions with your friends makes the experience easier. Before you know it you will have created a habit and it will not even feel like exercise anymore.

Beth

# PART SEVEN

# HEALTH CONCERNS

I have yet to meet anyone fifty years and older who has absolutely no health concerns or joint problems. Oftentimes there is an old sports injury that causes us to experience some sort of pain when we move a certain way. Maybe we are carrying quite a bit of weight around the middle from either poor eating habits or from lack of movement which limits our ability to participate fully in activities that used to bring us joy. Many of my clients, of all different ages, suffer from some type of arthritis which flares up from time to time. My point is we all have some sort of issue that we need to address and most of my clients use fitness as a way to manage their personal situation.

I have so many inspiring stories of people overcoming their health challenges through regular attendance in my classes but one of the best perspectives comes from Mariette. She used to attend classes in my home studio before COVID and she is one of my longest attending members. Whenever it was time to register, she would remind those who questioned her commitment that she prefers to pay me to keep her in good health, instead of paying for medicine.

Now some of us need to take medication to manage our disease even when exercising but in most cases regular physical activity allows us to decrease our dependence on pain relievers and other drugs.

I hope that the following section helps you to realize that you are not alone.

# PLEASE TELL ME

March 1, 2017

Please remember that your safety is my number one priority and it's very important that you share certain health information with me, so that I can guide you through to a successful workout.

A few weeks ago, one of my strongest students suffered a serious fall while walking to class. They slipped on the ice and fell backwards onto the sidewalk. Luckily, the backpack that they were wearing saved them from a serious crack on the skull. This student was right to tell me about the accident before beginning the class because I was able to offer advice and check on them throughout the hour-long session.

Last Monday, a second student slipped in the parking lot and hit their head. This person only told me about the incident after the class. When I told them that that was not a good idea, the student explained that they had mentioned their fall to a fellow participant. While this is better than nothing, keep in mind that should you pass out, that person may fail to let me know what had happened to you only minutes before. I need to know about these situations, so that I can fully inform any medical team who arrive on the scene. It is just common sense.

Last year, one of my older participants was experiencing occasional paralysis in one leg. They did not mention this to me for fear of not being allowed to continue classes and as a result, they fell during the cardio component and almost injured others in the process. Had I been informed, I would have selected a different warm up for this student to keep everyone safe.

Just yesterday, a client who had suffered a serious fall and head injury when they fell down some stairs the night before, only told me about the accident after the cardio portion of the class. I noticed a large bruise and asked some questions.

Falls of this nature are very serious. You may have a concussion or a serious neck injury and I need to know this so that I can make recommendations on how to proceed safely with your exercise session. If nothing else, I will at least pay more attention to your posture and demeanor and be able to act quickly if a serious situation arises.

Remember that we are a team on your journey towards better health. Please let me know if you have fallen recently. I want to keep you safe.

Sincerely,

Beth

# TAKE NOTE OF PHYSICAL CHANGES

December 2, 2015

I have often remarked about how strong my students are. I know that many of you are battling various conditions and yet you still manage to get yourself to class and smile! I am inspired every day by your courage and your resilience.

Today's message is just a wee reminder to listen to your body and to take note of little changes you may notice in your physical wellbeing. Perhaps you are experiencing bouts of dizziness due to a medication change or maybe you are finding yourself short of breath during mild activity. Your trainer or instructor needs to know about these changes in order to keep you safe during your exercise sessions and these indicators should lead to adaptations in your workout.

There is a tendency among students to want to continue doing the same class, exactly the same way, despite these changes. I totally understand the desire to cling to our routines, however it is very important to speak to the instructor and let them know what is going on regarding your health. If you are in my classes, I will do my best to suggest alternative exercises to help you adapt to these changes in your health or I may advise a short time of rest.

Your health and safety is my ultimate concern. We have to work together to keep you fit!

Beth

# IS YOUR POOR POSTURE MAKING YOU SICK?

May 25, 2015

If you have been in my class than you are aware of how often I ask you to be mindful of your posture. If you exercise with poor posture you will get hurt over time, so I am constantly reminding everyone to maintain proper form and technique. In fact, this is why I end many of my classes with a upward stretch, saying, "Take a deep breath in, reaching your arms up, making yourself taller than you were when you came in!" I am trying to combat the ill effects of computer and cell phone activities.

Last week, I visited my physio because of some shoulder pain I was experiencing. After a proper evaluation she found that the problem was coming from my neck. I will spare you the details but I spend a fair amount of time working on my laptop and my cell phone which causes my neck to move in front of my shoulders. Dr. Travis McDonough, explains that this posture can lead to the following health problems:

* For every half an inch that the head moves in front of the shoulder, this increases the weight of the head by 20 pounds. This can lead to neck pain, jaw problems and headaches, all of which I have had lately.

* In this rounded position we compress the chest which makes it harder to breathe. In order to breathe in this position, we have to raise our shoulders to allow the diaphragm to go down. When we do this with each breath, it leads to tightness and tension in the upper back and neck. I have had a few young people lately tell me they sometimes feel like they are having a heart attack because their chest feels so tight and hurts to breathe. In their case it was all related to poor posture.

*Our vertebrae are meant to stack on top of each other and when we assume this hunched position over time, the vertebrae at the front get compressed and this can lead to 'Dowager's Hump' or a hunched back. It is most often associated with the elderly but in my work, I am seeing it manifest much earlier. Have a look at yourself in the mirror as you stand sideways. Stand normally. Is your upper back rounded and are you starting to see a 'hump?' None of us want this. Keeping your back straight will help you to avoid this.

* Shoulder problems can become quite serious when we assume this hunched over position as the muscles in our chest get tight and the muscles in the back get loose. This imbalance can lead to rotator cuff injuries which are very painful, and costly to remedy with physio or surgery.

How can we fix this problem right now?

Dr. McDononough suggests the following to minimize the impact:

* Move the chin back to its natural position over the spine and then pretend you are balancing a book on top of your head. Do this for three seconds and then relax. Repeat.

* Squeeze the shoulder blades together and then relax. Repeat.

I recommend that if you spend most of your day on the computer, get up every 20 minutes and walk around. Do the above exercises and resume your activities. Try to keep the head and shoulders back. I hope these tips help you to avoid injury and pain.

Beth

# ESSENTRICS® CAN HELP

January 4, 2018

Are you tired of stiff joints? Sore neck muscles? Painful knees and hips? I believe that the Essentrics® full body workout may be able to alleviate your discomfort because this program re-balances all 600 + muscles in the body.

After the long holiday break most of us are feeling stiff because of inactivity. We can also feel stiff from not using all of our muscles daily. We really do 'lose it' if we do not use it. None of our body parts are optional and each one needs to be moved the way it was designed to move or it stops functioning properly. This can lead to pain and immobility. I am thinking of those clients who avoid certain actions because "they just cannot do it anymore." Perhaps Essentrics® can help.

Most of the time we focus on certain body parts or components of fitness in our various classes together because it is almost impossible to get to everything in the one hour. Well Miranda Esmonde-White has designed her Essentrics® program to combat the muscle imbalances often created by traditional training methods.

I started my training to become an Essentrics® instructor in October. I began teaching apprentice classes in my home and in the homes of friends and family last November and I am truly amazed at the changes in my body. While I was in pretty good shape when I began, I doubted whether the program would impact my health personally, simply because I believed that I had seen it all! Much to my surprise my arms are stronger and more defined to the point where someone asked me last week, "How do I get arms like yours?" In 20 years of teaching, no one has ever asked me that so I attribute it to Essentrics®. I no longer have lingering back pain from an old injury years ago. Over the last year, I had been experiencing some bursitis in my hip on and off but since I began Essentrics®, the pain has stopped completely. I feel taller and thinner in my mid-section and more flexible than ever before!

Keep in mind that we do not lift any weights in this type of class. We do not hold postures for long periods of time which can have a negative impact on painful joints. In fact we move continually throughout the workout along the body's natural chains of movement. This is part of the reason that you will leave a class feeling refreshed and energized and even taller!

I have been very busy over the holiday break completing my training. I am awaiting my certification in the mail. It is a rigorous training process and very rewarding. I cannot wait to share Essentrics® with you in the coming year!

Beth

# DO NOT BECOME THE DISEASE

May 27, 2015

Osteopenia. Osteoporosis. Arthritis. Diabetes. Heart Disease. High Blood Pressure. Cancer.

If you suffer from one of these conditions, my guess is that you know how it feels to be told that you are not who you thought you were.... suddenly you have a disease!

Every month or so I have a student coming up to tell me that their doctor has told them that they have 'xyz.' I can see the look of sadness in their eyes. Some have cried. At times I have cried with them. Depending on the disease and the severity sometimes they have to stop exercising with me but in many cases, their doctor has told them that the exercise has prevented the condition from being worse and that the prescription is more exercise! No matter what the case, my message is always the same. You must listen to your body. When something feels wrong, you stop. You are the boss of you in my class and whatever your doctor or physiotherapist says is more important than anything you hear come out of my mouth.

Please remember that while you are fighting the condition, you are "NOT THE DISEASE." Yes, you have had to make adjustments. Yes, it has been hard but deep inside, you are still YOU.  Do not become the disease. Do not let it rob you and the rest of the world of your identity. The disease is just a tiny bit of you.

Whether you just found out or you have been struggling for awhile, you are an amazing person with huge potential while you are on this earth.

Beth

# DIZZINESS AFTER YOGA

June 24, 2015

In one of my yoga classes yesterday, I had a new student ask me if it was normal that she felt dizzy. The answer is yes. During yoga it is normal to experience some sort of physical release. As Beth Shaw explains in her book, *Yogafit*, we can experience nausea, lightheadedness, dizziness, muscle cramps, tingling sensations and flatulence. Hey, it happens!

In fact, all of these symptoms can be experienced during any form of physical exercise. This student in particular exercises regularly but this was her first yoga class so even if you are in shape, when you try something new, you can still have a physical release that is foreign to you. When the sensations are concerning like dizziness it is important to rest and not push yourself further. I tell students that during the class if I do anything that makes them uncomfortable to return to a resting position and just breathe. With continued practice, these sensations will usually disappear. As Beth explains they are often a result of a release in stress and tension.

As I have mentioned in previous blog posts, many of us are unaware that stress is impacting our health and it is only when we actually take the time to slow down and remember what being 'calm' actually feels like, that we notice the difference. Most of us are not breathing well during exercise or life in general. Our lungs have a huge capacity but we are only using the top third. Learning how to breathe deeply can also bring on some lightheadedness simply because you are not used to it. The only time you need to worry about the above symptoms is if they persist. Then you would need to ask your health care professional for further advice.

Beth

# IS RELAXATION HAZARDOUS TO OUR HEALTH?

August 1, 2016

I finally have proof that though I can teach fourteen hours of fitness a week, for twelve weeks straight, and never miss work, I often get sick when I stop! Many fitness instructors I know have experienced the same thing. Many people get sick in the middle of vacation and feel cheated.

According to Marc Schoen, PhD and author of *When Relaxation is Hazardous to Your Health*, a phenomenon called, the 'Let Down Effect' can result in us getting sick once we eliminate the stress of work or a big project.

When we are under stress, our body is equipped to fight for survival but if we come to a screeching halt and drop onto the couch for days, Dr. Schoen claims that this can "lead to biochemical changes that can result in a weakened immunity." I am happy to say that I have been quite healthy this summer because I kept five classes running, but even this small change resulted in a calf injury. I stopped my daily routine of stretching because I was no longer teaching yoga every day.

The best advice that I can give to avoid getting ill on vacation, is to keep doing a small portion of your fitness routine daily or weekly. It is so tempting to give in to our desire to do absolutely nothing. Many of my students continue to walk and stretch when they are cruises or tropical beach vacations. When I know that you are leaving on vacation for a few weeks, I tell you to walk and stretch daily and then I did not follow my own advice! I look forward to getting back to our workout schedule in September but until then keep as active as you can.

# DOES YOUR BACK HURT?

March 14, 2016

I have a few friends/clients who are currently experiencing back pain. Some of them have been to physiotherapy in the past for the same issue and they are doing their exercises at home as prescribed by their health care professional. Others have taken time off of work to rest and be able to go to physiotherapy two or three times a week. It is so important to listen to your body.

If you have ever had back pain you know how uncomfortable life can be. Just doing daily activities can be quite a chore. This past Friday, Dr. Oz did a segment to address the problem of long lasting back pain. So many people suffer with this that he had a physiotherapist come on and give some helpful tips. I am happy to say that the exercises she demonstrated are some of the exact ones that I do in my yoga stretch classes.

First, you must determine what the issue is with your back so that you do not make it worse. A qualified physiotherapist can tell you which movements to avoid, and what exercises you need to do to strengthen the weak muscles that added to your problem in the first place. I cannot stress the importance of a proper diagnosis enough! You do not want to aggravate the situation, you want relief. The following movements were shown on Dr.Oz and they happen to be a part of my classes. She suggested doing them before you get out of bed but most of us sleep with a partner, so this would be difficult for a lot of us. If any of these cause you pain, stop immediately and ask your physiotherapist if these exercises are safe for you.

1. While lying on your back, gently draw one knee into your chest, hold and release and repeat with the other leg. This loosens up the hamstrings and stretches the lower back. This

is the first motion that I do with my gentle yoga stretch classes. Do not forget to breathe.

2. Lie on your stomach with one hand under your chin and the other arm up beside your ear. Lift the opposite arm and leg and then repeat on the other side. We do this in class on all fours. This strengthens the back, butt and also stretches the front of the body. We inhale as we lift and exhale as we lower.

3. While lying on your back, with legs straight, raise one knee up until it is over the hip, push against the knee while resisting. Switch sides. Exhale as you push, inhale as you lower. Do not hold your breath. This exercise strengthens your abdominals without flexing your spine. We do a variation of this isometric work in class but I usually save this exercise for individuals suffering with pain who are in my Chair Muscle conditioning classes.

I hope that this will provide a bit of relief. It is nice to see that I am on the right track. Ultimately you have to listen to your own body and do what feels right for you!

Beth

# IS IT VERTIGO OR DIZZINESS? KNOW THE FACTS

November 3, 2020

I have suffered from positional vertigo so I know that there is a big difference between being dizzy (feeling lightheaded and off balance) to having your eyes spinning uncontrollably inside your head, where you feel like you are doing fast somersaults. You would not believe how often I have students show up in class and tell me that they are having a vertigo attack. I have learned that whether it is actually vertigo or dizziness, it is important to tell people to go at their own pace and stop if something feels wrong. I decided to ask Andrea Dewar, registered physiotherapist, and friend, to come and talk to my virtual studio members about the difference between the two conditions and here are the important points from her lecture last week.

The first message I want to get across was the last point that Andrea made. Staying in shape is your number one way to prevent these attacks from happening. We need to do both cardiorespiratory training and muscular conditioning as well as flexibility improvement exercises. Why? Because many cases of dizziness can be attributed to poor fitness and poor posture. If you never train your heart and lungs, you will not be able to nourish your body properly with oxygen, and if you also have weak postural muscles and carry a hunched back or vulture neck position all day long, your lungs are not able to expand fully. These two facts alone create a situation where you might become prone to breathing issues which can bring on dizziness issues. Stress management is also key because when we are tense, we tighten our neck muscles and cervical spine health becomes compromised so Andrea suggests that we practice deep breathing techniques, yoga or meditation to keep our stress levels under control.

How do you know the difference between simple dizziness and vertigo? Andrea explained the two as follows:

**DIZZINESS**: spatial orientation is off, usually characterized as a non-specific sensation (floating feeling, lightheadedness, unstable, feeling as if on a boat, feeling drunk). This feeling can be brought on by lying to sitting or standing, coming back up from squatting low down, standing for long periods of time without moving. We can experience blurred vision, feel faint, feel pressure in the head and even see rings of light.

**VERTIGO**: defined by a sensation of rotatory movement, spinning or turning. Can be both a feeling that the environment around is turning or spinning (external) or that one feel themselves turning around 360 degrees. In my case, my eyes cannot focus and I feel as though I am physically doing fast somersaults.

The next important take away is that if you are experiencing any dizziness, to go and see your doctor because it could be a sign of something more serious.

For example, feeling faint could mean that there is something wrong with your heart. Feeling unstable or wobbly could mean that your muscles are deconditioned or that the natural degeneration of the inner ear has progressed to such a rate as to affect your balance. Medications can make us feel off balance too. Concussions can bring on dizziness as well as tightness in the neck muscles. Andrea also pointed out that anemia and hypoglycemia can also contribute to sensations of dizziness. The clear message here is you have to see a medical professional to rule out serious health problems. I always tell you to listen to your body. It is telling you something.

**VERTIGO causes:**

1. **Benign Positional Paroxysmal vertigo (BPPV) – What is it?**

- Tiny crystals that are located in one area of your inner ear (utricle) get dislodged and migrate into the semicircular canals of the inner ear. Incidence increases after 55 years of age. Ratio of women to men is 2:1

- Idiopathic 60-80% of the time. Can be related with Osteoporosis, Osteopenia, auto-immune diseases, diabetes, anxiety.

- 10-30% of BPPV are caused by trauma

- 5-25% of BPPV are caused by other illnesses (upper respiratory track are very common)

**BPPV Symptoms** can give us a feeling of intense VERTIGO that lasts from seconds to maximum one minute and are related with quick changes in the position of the head

\* Usually dizziness, nausea and balance isues follows the vertigo sensation and can last for

hours afterwards

\* People end up avoiding the movement that provoked the vertigo.

## 2. Labyrinthitis:

- Virus or a bacterial infection of the ear

- Temporary altered hearing of the ear affected

- If bacterial treated with antibiotics

- Acute vertigo typically lasts less than 24 hours

- Balance affected, eyes affected (Nystagmus), nausea, symptoms can last up to three months

- Often treated with antivertigo meds in acute cases like Teva Beta Histine (SERC), Gravol

## 3. Vestibular Neuritis

- Viral Infection affecting Vestibular nerve

- Severe vertigo lasting typically less than 48 hours

- No auditory symptoms

- Treated often with Gravol in ER (IV)
- Symptoms can last up to six weeks

**4. Serious head traumas**

 * Fractures of skull, concussions, scuba diving incidents.

**5. Meniere's disease**

 *Auto immune disease

 * Women 30-40 years old

 * Pressure builds in ear

 * Vertigo 20 minutes to a few hours

 * Re-occurring episodes over a ten-year span, ENT

 * Treated with medications (SERC, Gravol, limited salt intake, diuretic), injections or surgery in serious cases.

**6. Other potential causes of vertigo:**

- Acoustic neuromas (Schwannoma)
- Tumors of the brain
- Meningitis
- Alcohol
- Vitamin B12 deficiency
- Vertebral basilar insufficiency
- Vestibular Migraines
- Strokes
- Multiple Sclerosis

If you are experiencing any of the above symptoms you would first go to your doctor and if referred to a physio, Andrea would do a complete Vestibular Physio Evaluation to determine if it is dizziness or vertigo. She then walked us through the steps she uses to determine this and left us with some good news. If it is indeed BPPV vertigo it is the most common type, and the easiest to fix. Andrea now sees three or four patients a day with this condition. This is the type of vertigo that I suffer from and thankfully Andrea has taught me how to manage it.

BVVP is a mechanical problem and moving the head in the right sequence can put the ear crystals back into the right place. Once you know in which of the six canals the crystals are located, Andrea then has specific maneuvers that will stop the spinning sensation. The bad news is that there is an 80% chance of reoccurrence within the first year. I have had three attacks since my first in the spring of 2019.

Andrea explained that she suffered from an attack of **viral** vertigo which was far more serious. The spinning took place for 24 hours and she had to be hospitalized, so you need to see the doctor first to get the proper diagnosis. I do not recommend doing any of the maneuvers on your own without seeing a specialist first because you could make your situation worse. However, Andrea gave us detailed descriptions of the Epley and the Semont maneuvers. I am able to remedy my vertigo with the right Semont maneuver.

If you want to discuss your dizziness with Andrea Dewar, she can be found at the Action Sport Physio Clinic in either Vaudreuil or Pointe Claire and she also has an office in her home. I highly recommend booking an appointment today. Don't suffer needlessly. Get informed and hopefully you will be moving normally once again with no dizzy feelings!

Beth

# CAN SOMEONE WITH ARTHRITIS DO ESSENTRICS?

February 7, 2018

In her most recent book, *Forever Painless,* Miranda explains that Essentrics® can help relieve the pain associated with arthritis because "it strengthens the muscles in a lengthened position, literally pulling the joints apart" (Esmonde-White, 2016, p. 233). It is this separating of the joints that provides pain relief because the bones stop grinding upon one another. While regular passive stretching can provide some relief, what is really needed is the strengthening of the muscles in the lengthened position so that they can properly support the joint and keep it decompressed.

There are many different forms of Arthritis and each individual suffers to differing degrees. I have several students who tell me that they must keep exercising or their joints stiffen up completely. Whenever they are in a flare up, they have been told by their doctor to avoid pushing through pain. I have always told my students to stop immediately if they feel intense pain. Your body is speaking to you and you must listen. Some days are better than others so if you are in this situation move gently and be kind to yourself.

In Essentrics® we move slowly compared to other workouts and we move through the whole muscle chain in order to work in a balanced fashion. This 'slowness' is perfect for allowing each individual the opportunity to gauge the suitability of the exercise for them specifically, on any given day. What worked for you last week may be too hard today but that does not mean that you need to give up entirely.

I have been getting wonderful feedback from the students in my Essentrics® classes. One lady confessed to me this week that she no longer wants to go to her yoga class. She just wants to do Essentrics® all of the time. I am starting to feel the same way. I absolutely love teaching this technique. Even though I only started doing this workout last October, my body craves the sensation of feeling totally stretched and strong at the same time. I walk away from my mat feeling completely energized. It is a wonderful feeling.

Essentrics® can be adapted to help you to manage your arthritis. Please speak to me if you would like some more information or support.

Beth

# FOCUS ON WHAT YOU CAN DO!

February 8, 2017

I know a few people this winter who are either recovering from an injury or facing surgery to repair a problem. I also know of at least two students who have broken an arm or a wrist because they suffered a fall. One client who recently joined my class is there because the doctor told her to build up her muscles before she has hip surgery. She cannot be more than 55 or 60 years old. I know that many of these people are feeling down because their situation is getting in the way of their regular routines.

I think that we can all agree that the only constant is change. We get depressed when we want things to stay the same. I have had my own physical challenges over the years. I went through a period of time when I had to limit my dancing due to foot pain. I am still dancing but I had to make adjustments to my routine. And because of my gluten allergy, I can no longer eat as freely as I once did.

My message today is there is joy on the other side of change if we focus on finding solutions that keep us moving forward. If you are faced with a physical challenge, focus on what you can do at this time, instead of what you can't. Chances are you can still exercise but you might have to switch to something that is easier on your joints. Perhaps you have to stop doing some things that you love for a short period of time while your body heals but you find that you love those new activities! I myself have learned to love food again by being open to eating differently.

There really is no point in mourning what we have lost. Try to be positive in the face of this new challenge. Explore new opportunities and you will find your groove once again.

# HOW MUCH DO YOU WORRY?

August 5, 2015

I am very guilty of worrying too much. I have a feeling that I am not alone. We are conditioned to worry. The news that we watch every day, tells us about things that are happening in the world, which we can do very little about. Tragedies of all kinds fill our thoughts, as we get ready to head out into the world for the day. I am certain that this adds to our daily stress levels.

I wonder what our experience in the world would be like if we saw as many positive news stories as negative ones. I know that the news I watch tries to throw in one 'feel good' story every broadcast but what if it was a 50/50 split of good news and bad news? I have a feeling that our worrying would stop and that our view on life would instantly improve.

My message today is that a constant pattern of worrying can directly impact our health. We are being bombarded by bad news all day long and as a result, we tend to think the worst when it comes to our own situations. It has become common to search the internet when we get diagnosed with a problem and that can lead us to imagining that our case is as bad as the most extreme news stories that we find on the web! It is incredibly hard to stay positive when we are facing a health challenge.

If you are struggling with something, sit for a minute and think of how far you have come. Focus on one positive accomplishment, no matter how small and take it from there. Speak to your health care professionals and remember that the particulars of your situation are unique and manageable with the right tools and attitude. Let's not get caught up in endless worry. Reach out for help and get the facts. Then keep your attitude as positive as possible.

# ARE YOU LISTENING TO YOUR BODY?

October 4, 2017

"If I listened to my body, I'd never get off my butt and come to class!" I overheard a student say this last week and I laughed quite hard. I always tell my students to listen to the signs that their body might be giving them so that they don't ignore pain and hurt themselves while training. However, some people live in chronic pain so they have to figure out when the pain is tolerable so they can workout on those days.

Yesterday a client admitted to me that she had been feeling chest pain that was not going away so she went to the hospital in fear that she might be having a heart attack. After all of the tests the doctors told her that it was muscular. I am glad that she got it checked out and I am glad that she is alright. It is better to be safe, than sorry. What concerns me are the little injuries that people ignore that can then turn into bigger problems. If you after class you feel pain in part of your body that you have never felt before, it is far better to go and see a physiotherapist instead of waiting for it to go away on its own.

In most cases the physio can tell you what movement caused the pain and what to do to remedy the situation. The truth is we are aging every day and the situations of our lives are changing as well, which put stress on our bodies in all forms. We are in a constant state of flux and as such we need to pay attention to sudden headaches, knee, neck and back pain. I know of several students who cannot join us right now because they ignored early signs from their body. The good news is that if you deal with the situation early enough, you will be back to yourself in no time. We only have one body and it needs both exercise and loving attention. Please take care of yourselves!

Beth

# DO I EXERCISE WHEN IN PAIN?

February 23, 2016

I get asked this question quite frequently for two specific reasons.

Arthritis sufferers who live with chronic pain, realize that even when they are struggling they need to move or they will feel worse. The trick for this clientele is knowing when to take a rest day and when they should push themselves a bit to work out. I always tell my clients to first follow the doctor's orders and then to listen to their heart. It would not be right for me to insist that this type of client force themselves through a painful workout, when they may be in a flare up that could make their condition worse.

The other reason that I get asked if we should move when in pain, is when people have trained really hard at the gym and their muscles are so sore that they have trouble participating in activities of daily living. This type of discomfort can be normal up to three days after a hard workout. The key in this situation is to know the difference between injury and muscle fatigue.

For example, if when you push on the area in question and it is extremely painful, red and tender you may have an injury. If your whole thigh muscle simply feels sore this is usually a sign of muscle fatigue and therefore movement is encouraged. Taking a gentle yoga class and/or stretching will eliminate this type of soreness.

It always feels better to move than to sit and feel miserable and focus on our pain. Just choose the type of activity that feels right for you at the time and get moving.

Beth

# IN SHAPE AND STILL GOT SICK!

February 21, 2018

This week two of my students, who attend classes regularly, learned that despite years of training they may be facing disease. I can hear those who don't work out ready with their defense. "You see, he or she ate well, exercised daily in a gym, didn't smoke or drink and they still got sick! Why bother exercising?"

As we know there are no guarantees in life. The reason that I myself decided to hit the gym over 25 years ago was that my parents both lived with heart disease, and I wanted to do everything I could to avoid suffering the same fate. I fell in love with aerobics and before I knew it I had signed up to become a fitness instructor.

It's definitely heart breaking to learn that something is wrong with our body when we work so hard to protect it but I want my students to remember that because you have chosen to strengthen your muscles, improve your flexibility and your endurance, you are better equipped to face these health challenges. You have prepared your body for battle. Your heart and muscles are well tuned and ready to beat the disease.

What I know for sure is that the students who are already in shape recover much faster than those who have never put their bodies to the test. You are used to discomfort because of training. You are better able to face adversity because you know your body so well. Your body is used to the cycle of repair and recovery. You know that pain is temporary and can be beat with the proper mental attitude. Stay positive. I am proud of you and know that you will handle this new challenge to the best of your ability because of your dedication to fitness.

Beth

# WHEN IN DOUBT, CHECK IT OUT

September 16, 2016

Sometimes we simply feel off. We do not feel like ourselves and we push this sensation aside and blame it on all sorts of things. A change in our sleep, our diet or our workout regime. Please  go and see a doctor if you cannot pinpoint the problem.

One of my clients who I had not seen in over a year, returned yesterday to tell me why she had been absent for so long. It turns out that she had been in a car accident.  She was unharmed in the accident but people insisted she go and get checked out.  In the process they discovered that she had tumors in her lymph nodes.  Luckily she underwent surgery and therapy and she is fine today, but had she not gone to get checked out, I could be telling a very different story. This woman had no prior symptoms.  The car accident turned out to be a blessing.

When in doubt, we really have to defer to the experts and get checked out. If you are fit and in shape and still find yourself feeling unwell, go and visit the doctor.

Take care and see you soon,

Beth

# MAKE YOUR BODY YOUR BUSINESS

August 10, 2015

This weekend, I had the pleasure of visiting with an old friend whom I had not seen in a long time. As he was walking toward me, I commented on how slow and cautious he was walking. He is 45 and as such, should be full of energy. It turns out that his old knee injury has come back to haunt him and he is looking at having surgery to repair the problem. To add to that, he now has a shoulder problem.

I am not without problem areas of my own. If we have been on this planet long enough, most of us develop some sort of injury through daily living or repetitive motions in our jobs. My message to you today is that simply being mildly active, walking the dog etc. is not enough to keep your joints in good shape. The muscles and tendons and ligaments that surround the joints of your body need to be trained equally to keep everything moving properly. You many not notice anything at the moment but do not wait until you have an injury to find out that you have imbalances.

I have been through many sessions of physiotherapy and what I have learned is that the muscle imbalances that we create through the job that we choose or the sports that we play etc., can cause us to have serious injuries later on in life. The physiotherapist then recommends exercises that will correct the problem. Why not do it the other way around? Get into the gym and address your imbalances on your own time, instead of it being forced on you because of a painful injury that is keeping you from your job and the activities that you love. The choice is ours!

I work with clients from the ages of 17-90 years old and as such I see into the future. I can see the difference between people who have been working out in the gym, training all of their muscles properly versus those who have simply been mildly active.

Hire a reputable trainer. Spend a few hours learning how you can make your potential weak areas stronger. Be proactive instead of reactive. Don't wait for injury to force you into the gym.

Learning how to weight train to keep your muscles strong will not result in you looking like a body builder unless you want it to. Some people are afraid of this and avoid weights altogether. Lifting weights (five to eight pounds) properly will keep your shoulders strong. Doing abdominal exercises will help to prevent future back problems. Doing push-ups and back extensions (superman) will keep your chest and back happy. Training all of the muscles equally around your knee joint with squats, lunges and inner and outer thigh work, will help to prevent knee issues.

Make your body your business and take your physical conditioning seriously to avoid future visits to the physiotherapist.

Beth

# EXERCISE AS INSURANCE

April 26, 2017

My struggle as a trainer is trying to convince people that they need to exercise for tomorrow, when today their health seems just fine. We need to start looking at exercise as insurance against the threats that exist to our health. We all buy car and house insurance just in case something terrible happens, so that we will be covered and better able to handle the situation. It is the same for exercise. Making sure that your body is in top shape will ensure that your body is better able to handle any issues that come your way.

I learned last week that one of my neighbours had a stroke a few months ago. He is in his early sixties. He is paralyzed on one side of the body and unable to speak. This has been bothering me ever since I learned the news because over ten years ago, I pleaded with him to start exercising. I could see the toll that work stress was taking on his body but he saw no need to fit fitness into his busy life.

I know that there are no guarantees that exercise will prevent us from getting sick or injured, but I know that your recovery time will be shorter and easier if you head into stressful situations in good physical condition.

The time to start exercising is when you think you don't need it or when you feel you have no time. Chances are you are physically able to join classes at the gym and all you need to do is organize your time better to take care of yourself.

Let's do this!

Beth

# YES, I AM LIKE YOU

May 25, 2016

When I meet people outside of the gym and tell them what I do for a living, often the first thing that they do is tell me the state of their health. I once ran into an acquaintance at the grocery store and she immediately started justifying all of the food within her cart. Then there are the folks who pretend that they want to exercise and inquire about my fees and ask for my business card. Nine times out of ten, I never hear from them. When I am off duty, as in not in the gym, I am not looking to judge anyone. I want you to know that I eat junk food. I have bad days and days when I don't want to work out. I continue to struggle with many of the same issues as you do. The point is I can see a bit of myself in every person.

I too have gained unwanted weight and I know how hard it is to lose it in a society that socializes around food. I know all the excuses to avoid exercise because I have made many of them myself. I know that life is busy and that it is hard to get to the gym but I also know the signs of people who have given up on themselves. I know that the last thing that you want is to become a burden to your friends and family. I know that if you loved yourself more, you would address the issues that are keeping you from taking better care of yourself. I know that you need someone to tell you that you are worth it!

You deserve to live a healthy life. Your family is counting on you to be there to help them navigate this world. They need you to be in the best shape that you can be. If you will not do it for yourself, do it for them and know that I am here to support you in any way that I can because I am just like you!

Beth

# PART EIGHT
# MENTAL HEALTH AND WELLNESS

If there is one thing that I know for sure after so many years of working in the fitness business, exercise helps us to feel better mentally. Without getting into the science behind the hormones that are released, I think we can all agree that though it can be hard at times, we rarely regret walking, biking, swimming or skiing. While the exercise might be challenging, it almost always leaves us feeling more alive than when we started, with a clearer mind and a happy heart.

I can remember my very first aerobics class. I had had our first child and was feeling tired, fat and slightly depressed. I knew that I had to lose the baby weight, so I did what most folks do, I signed up for an exercise class. I had tried jazz ballet when I was an awkward teenager, and though I was concerned that I would look just as lost as I did back then, I knew that this aerobics class was the key to me feeling better emotionally. The teacher was energetic, and the music was fun and inspiring. Yes, I stumbled all over the place, but for that one hour I had to focus on something else, so my mind got a break from the worry while the benefits of physical exercise took place.

As an instructor I can easily recognize when someone is overwhelmed by life. Oftentimes my students are the primary caregiver for their ailing spouse or parent. One client in particular used to arrive several minutes late to class, which tends to bother other students, but I knew that she had to drop off her husband (who suffers from Alzheimer's) at a daycare center in order to be able to take care of her own health.

My primary goal is to encourage exercise of any kind and because I know that everyone is carrying unique responsibilities, my job as your trainer is to do all I can to offer an empathetic, supportive environment that is ready to welcome you whenever you can make time for yourself.

When it comes to battling mental health issues, the greatest advice that I can give you is make exercising as easy and automatic as possible. Sign up for a workout that takes place at the same time each day and plan ahead by telling your family and friends that you are committed to taking care of yourself at that hour. Lay out your clothes and shoes and gear the night before. Set a timer to remind you of class and turn the notifications off on your phone. Be fully present and allow the teacher to lead your body through the movements and in the process, your mental health will improve over time. Fitness really is a cure for most of what ails us.

Please reach out if I can offer any extra support. I am always here for you.

# A MESSAGE OF HOPE

September 12, 2019

There's always something you can do, even when you think you can't. My students have taught me this lesson time and time again. My message today: you are stronger than you realize!

If you're feeling beaten down by life's challenges or by a physical ailment, moving and exercise will help. Pumping blood throughout the body delivers fresh oxygen and healing nutrients to the muscles and tissues. Walking, dancing, and stretching clear the mind and help us to focus on something outside of ourselves and that is when the magic happens. You see, for the most part I'm preoccupied with teaching an effective, safe program to my students but once the class is rolling along smoothly, I get to see how people are adapting the exercises to suit their personal situation and it inspires me.

Stroke patients who use a chair but do 90% of the class like the rest of us have proven to me that moving is essential to good health. Arthritis sufferers who move a bit slower, with no resistance, usually walk away from class feeling better than when they walked in. People struggling with negative emotions find themselves smiling a bit more.

Please listen to your health care professional and follow their advice but remember that we are more resilient than we realize. Don't let anyone else put limits on your potential. There is always something you can do toward healing yourself. I look forward to another great year of being inspired by my students!

Beth

# CONFRONT YOUR ISSUES WITH ACCEPTANCE

February 18, 2016

Yoga-inspired workouts are a great place for self evaluation. Discovering that you cannot touch your toes like someone else your age or older is a sobering experience. Discovering that your wrists, knees or your hips are too tight to hold certain poses with any degree of confidence or comfort, can be quite discouraging. Past injuries can make certain poses completely unattainable. Confronting these issues is part of learning acceptance, for who we are, at that very moment.

We cannot change the things that happen to us but we can change our reaction. Instead of beating ourselves up for not being able to do perfect poses, yoga affords us the time and space in which we can learn to relax into who we are today. If we wish to improve our physical or mental state, yoga can help us to do so at our own pace, whether this means becoming more flexible or simply accepting our limitations. Let's face it having limited flexibility is stressful on our joints. Not being able move with ease can cause us to avoid living. Perhaps we do not participate in family activities because of various physical limitations. This stress can erode our health in more ways than one.

I remind my students that even though we may experience challenges during certain poses, learning to simply breathe and accept, ultimately teaches us how to deal with stress better in our daily lives. All that matters is our ability to breathe in and breathe out. Yoga practice is a great place to start accepting and loving ourselves.

Beth

# WHERE IS YOUR SUPPORT?

March 29, 2017

Feeling healthy is not just about watching our weight. We can be the correct weight for our height and have strong, flexible muscles and great cardiovascular stamina, and still feel unwell. We also need to take care of our mental health. How are you feeling emotionally? Do you feel heard? Do you feel lonely? Sometimes these feelings can stand in the way of us achieving our goals.

I have written to you before about how important it is for us to feel supported by our families and friends. Last year, I was lucky enough to be invited to join a Women's Circle that was starting up in Montreal. This circle is different from a group of friends meeting over coffee. We meet every two weeks and we take turns speaking from our heart, no matter what is on our mind. We do not comment on what was said just before and when it is not our turn, we remain quiet and only listen. The idea is to express our feelings without fear of judgement.

It is an exercise in listening and the benefits are many because not only do you get a chance to talk about what is on your mind, you are not interrupted when you are speaking, which sometimes happens in regular conversation. By the end of your turn, you feel as though you have genuinely been heard and that you have clearly expressed what is on your mind, to the point where you can now stop overthinking. You often hear yourself coming through in what everyone else is saying, so you learn time and time again that we are not alone and that we all feel the same things. Whatever is said in the circle, remains in the circle. The most important part of the group is privacy. You have to trust.

Clients often ask me why they are not losing weight or achieving their fitness goals. The truth is I can make adjustments to your program and I can advise you to eat well and get plenty of quality sleep, but the answer may rest in how you are feeling emotionally. We have to treat the body as a whole. Unresolved feelings may be causing you to make bad choices when it comes to eating and drinking, and/or stress may be undermining your weight loss goals. If our minds are filled with worry our physical self suffers.

Joining a supportive group of women was the best decision I have made in a long time. Though it was a group of complete strangers one year ago, today I consider them to be some of my closest friends. I hope that you can surround yourself with support. Reach out if you need help.

Beth

# I SEE YOU!

May 17, 2017

I teach several classes and see over 100 students a day. I do my best to connect with as many people as I can while delivering quality programming, in a timely manner. Most of my classes are fifty-five minutes long and back to back, so there is not a lot of time for personal conversations but I do my best to make myself available to those students with burning questions or comments. My message today is simple. I see you even though I may not be able to talk with you personally.

I see the progress that you are making in your fitness training but I also notice when you are tired or feeling down. Most of the time my students give off a positive energy and everyone is happy to be together but there are days when the energy is low and often this is connected to global events or local news items. My challenge is to avoid soaking up negative vibes like a sponge because this makes it harder for me to lift your spirits and help you to get fit. Please know that at times I have to maintain some distance so that I get you to leave your worries behind and focus on the task at hand – getting fit!

The greatest gift that you can give to yourself when you are training is to focus solely on the moment. Focus on your breath, your posture and the mechanics of the exercise. When the class is over, you will feel refreshed and hopefully energized differently than when you walked in. I see you and I hear you and I am grateful for your presence. Thank you for trusting me with your fitness.

Beth

# COGNITIVE DECLINE IS REAL!

February 26, 2020

I am on the front lines. I see first hand how my students have changed over the last five years in their ability to process instructions in a timely, correct manner. I don't mean to be an alarmist but the bells are ringing. It is time to put more attention on challenging your mind.

I try my best to adjust my programming to suit the needs of my many students. I now see that I need to add more mental stimulus to our workouts to try to mitigate the problem, but my question to you today is a simple one: what are you doing when we are not together to challenge your mind?

I encourage you to put as much focus on keeping your mind sharp as you do on attending the gym every day for your muscles and bones. There are many games out there to keep your mind sharp and you can go the traditional route with board games or use your electronic devices. Most of you are in amazing physical shape and I want your mind to keep up with your body! Use it or lose it. I see several people in my line of work who are *losing it* far too young. Get busy.

One of the common complaints that I have heard over the years is, "I don't know my left from my right!" While this is a cute way to tell others not to follow you in class, I see the effect of people refusing to try to fix this with a concerted effort. Losing direction in class can be dangerous, especially in aerobics or dance class but if we ignore this, it can impact our driving ability and put others at risk on the road.

In many of my classes, I have to keep the movements quite simple because so many people are having trouble with multi-tasking and direction. When I give you directions in class, repeat them in your mind while doing them, and this will help reinforce your sense of direction and hopefully improve your ability to process the information.

It is quite normal for reaction time to slow down as we age but we can slow this effect by continually challenging our nervous system through targeted exercise. Eye hand co-ordination games like Pickle Ball and Tennis and Badminton all help to keep our reflexes sharp. Why is this important? As an instructor, I want you to be able to slow your body down in a fall. I want you to be able to catch yourself before hitting the ground, by getting a leg out in front of you fast enough but you need to practice these movements in a safe setting. You need to maintain flexibility and strength in your muscles to recover from being off balance and to withstand hitting the ground.

"But sports irritate my knees?" I can hear many of you saying this so here is my prescription. Seriously look into what is causing your knee pain. Spend the money to discuss your situation with a physiotherapist and then address the issue. Maybe you cannot take up Pickle Ball or Badminton, but then work hard to strengthen and stretch the imbalances around your knees because avoiding the issue will not make it go away. In a situation where you are falling, you need to have good flexibility and quick reflexes to avoid serious injury. I can't stress this enough. Once we pass 50 or 60 years of age, it takes longer to heal if we are not in good shape before an injury and often an injury will set us back in more ways than one. So let's address the issues that are keeping us from staying agile and be proactive instead of simply reactive.

Often, we stop moving to avoid pain in our joints but this is a dangerous cycle because the lack of movement results in atrophied weak muscles, which results in imbalances and sets us up for injury. Remember that we are fighting decay. A "rolling stone gathers no moss." We need to keep moving, in every way that our joints are designed to move, and we need to use our mind in the process. We are aging but we can ease the process through activities that challenge every aspect of our physical well being.

*"What a bummer blog post Beth!"*

Sorry everyone. I am here to keep it real. Remember, I need you guys to keep going so I can keep doing what I love.

Beth

# S.A.D? EXERCISE MIGHT NOT BE ENOUGH

January 22, 2020

Every winter I struggle with feeling down and I know that it's not because I need to exercise! Often doctors describe fitness for people who are depressed as a way of increasing energy and endorphins. I completely agree that exercise is the best medicine but it might not be the only solution for people who suffer with Seasonal Affective Disorder.

In my case, I'm active over 11 hours a week. I know that teaching dance and fitness helps me to feel happier, however I'm an early riser by nature and waking up to darkness really has a negative impact on my energy for the rest of the day. You see I'm most energetic between the hours of five and seven in the morning. This is when I write and do my creative arts and I just lose all momentum with no sunlight, so this year I took matters into my own hands and bought a therapy lamp.

I am not a doctor and I recommend seeking a professional opinion if you are feeling depressed but I am happy to report that this lamp has been a game changer for me after only one week of dedicated use. I rise early and turn on the lamp in my creative space. I make a cup of coffee (decaf) and walk back into my office now fully illuminated in bright light. I have the lamp on the windowsill to my left while I write and I never look directly at it but it mimics the sun and has resulted in me being more productive and as a consequence happier.

There are many different models but I chose one that has different shades and intensity options. It UV free and looks like a tablet. I tell others to get the proper tools for fitness that will help them to succeed, be it clothes, shoes, books or videos so

I needed to get myself a tool to help me to be at my best for my students. The best part is it is WORKING!

Beth

# TIPS TO BEAT THE WINTER BLUES

January 26, 2016

I feel it too. The darkness and the cold make it all too easy to want to curl up on the couch with a book and never go out. Okay, maybe I just feel this way! I couldn't even find a picture of myself outside in the winter to share with you.

I have spoken to a few people this January who have expressed a bit of sadness about the weather and how long winter can be in Quebec. One of my friends is really making a point of planning activities that keep her from hiding in her house waiting for spring. I am so proud of her. Maybe some of the following tips will help you to beat the winter blues.

* Try to find an art or a cooking class or join a book club or a bridge group that gets you out of the house a few times per week. Rather than taking a 'drop in' type class, try to find one that makes you register for the whole session. This will help you to stay committed. 'Dropping in' is just a way of planning to 'drop out' as far as I am concerned. Do yourself a favour and commit to being busy this winter.

* Several people I know volunteer their time to different organizations. This is a wonderful way to get out of the house and improve our mood by helping others. We also meet new people which can spur on even more activity.

* It is also very important to get out into the light and take in the sun. Light from the sun promotes the secretion of serotonin which increases positivity and alertness. Promise yourself that you will go for a short walk, every day out in the daylight.

* Fitness is very helpful at increasing energy levels. When we first start to train, exercise can be tiring but with a regular routine, you will find that you have more energy after class than you did when you arrived. Try to find a class that interests

you and then bring a friend. I find that students who plan to workout with a friend and then plan to visit afterwards, almost never miss class!

I am not a winter sport person. I do like to skate but usually the wind makes me retreat for hot chocolate shortly after lacing up my skates! Two or three times during the winter I follow my husband to the rink and we skate. I was far more active in the winter when my kids were little and I knew that I had to get them outside for fresh air. I used to spend hours sliding with my little ones.

Even though I do not like to play outside in the cold anymore, I am trying my best to have many activities that keep me distracted while winter moves along. At the beginning of the week, I try to make plans with friends for lunch or coffee so my week is filled with plans to get me out of the house.

I hope some of these tips help you to keep your smiles for the next two months. We can do this!

Just come to the gym if all else fails and I will get you sweating like it is full on summer!

Beth

# FEELING OVERWHELMED AND MISERABLE

May 12, 2016

I had two separate clients say to me this week, "I can't believe how hard I have had it this winter!" In both cases, the people have suffered either with illness or injury and one of the ladies has had several unexpected home repairs happening all at the same time. I can sympathize with each of them. It is amazing how some periods, months or years in our lives can seem so full of sorrow and strife.

One of my favourite books is called, *When Things Fall Apart*, by Pema Chodron. This book helped me to navigate some of the difficult periods in my life, when it appeared that everything was literally falling apart. Pema suggests that we "use difficult situations – as fuel for waking up."

Though it is hard at first, we can use these moments to develop a sense of empathy for others who are going through the very same difficulties. Instead of closing down into a 'woe is me' attitude, we can choose to focus on opening up to others and meditate on how all of us can be free from similar suffering. She sees this as the way to relieve our pain. It feels good to reach out to others who are suffering more than us and in so doing, we relieve our discomfort.

It sounds bizarre to even suggest focusing on others when we are suffering but I can remember being in the hospital, sitting by my dad's bedside and noticing that the lady beside him rarely had any visitors. There was a young man who sat in a chair reading the paper every once in a while but he did not engage with the lady at all, so I put myself in her shoes and wondered how badly she must be feeling. I started to chat with her and before you know it a beautiful smile appeared on her lips. I had been feeling weighed down by my own struggle but for that brief moment we both felt lighter.

Once we have lived through something challenging, we are forever able to recognize the look of a stranger facing similar situations. We are less judgmental because we can empathize with all that they may be going through. Putting ourselves in the other person's shoes takes practice but it helps me to remain open and kind.

Think back on one hard event that you have survived and remember those people who gave you a hand, a welcome smile or a nod of understanding. At that moment, they helped you to get through the day and their gestures were gifts. Hard times can harden us against the world or they can turn us into those little angels who offer smiles and hope.

If you feel that you are experiencing more than your fair share, perhaps you are being given these opportunities to turn your thinking around and make the world a better place.

Beth

# FOR KIDS AND ADULTS ALIKE

December 3, 2015

I am amazed how negative the news is of late. It would appear that the whole world has gone crazy and that we are all carrying guns or bombs, ready to annihilate anyone who disagrees with our world view. Yesterday, I listened to a social worker tell parents to turn off the television during the day, so that kids are not impacted by the negative images.

He was expressing how young children think that the images of the attack that took place days ago are happening again. They cannot distinguish the difference and because the news stations choose to show us the same violent images over and over again, this causes stress in little children because they think it is happening at this very moment. This may impact kids but I believe it impacts adults as well. I am convinced that all of us are negatively impacted by these reports that tell us stuff we already know, alongside horrible pictures that have been displayed a million times.

Be mindful about the amount of negative news that you are taking in, as it truly can make us unnecessarily fearful. Fear causes stress and too much stress can make us sick. Of course, we need to stay informed but do we really need to hear it over and over again? I think not. Consider what impacts your day the most and focus on knowing what you need to know, to go about your day. Let's focus our energy on leaving the space that we enter better than it was before we arrived! Share smiles with neighbours and friends and do your part to make the world a more positive place.

Beth

# WORDS ARE POWERFUL: USE THEM WISELY

May 16, 2018

We have all been in the position where a thought enters our head and we want to blurt it out to deliver a great punch line. It feels great to make a group of people smile or laugh when the comment is friendly and funny but even then, we really need to consider the impact that it might have on the group as a whole.

I often find myself in this position because I want to motivate my students and sometimes making them laugh goes a long way in helping clients push through the last reps of an exercise. There have been times when I have uttered things that were inappropriate and I have felt badly after class. It happens but I am proud to say that nine times out of ten, I use my words to encourage and support those around me in my classes and with my family and friends.

That is why I am surprised and caught off guard when someone makes a rude comment to me about my class. I work so hard to stop derogatory comments from popping out of my mouth that I choose to say nothing at all over risking offending someone. I am left speechless when someone offends me, because the thoughts that pile up on my tongue will cause more harm than good if I speak them aloud, so I keep my mouth shut.

This week someone was trying to be funny (I think) after I had finished teaching a class. I had not asked for any input but this person chose to speak out loudly in front of everyone, as they expressed their dissatisfaction with the class. People just ignored the comment because it was quite rude.

I want to let everyone know that teachers in general put many unpaid hours into learning their craft so that they can deliver the best classes possible. We stay up late studying and in my case, I spend hours buying new music and then countless hours practicing, so that I can lead my students through the workout or dance class safely while having fun at the same time! And in this process of learning some transitions will be smooth, while others will be bumpy.

I, like you, need time to get everything 'perfect.' Whatever that means...it is different for everyone!

When you see that a teacher is stepping out of their comfort zone, show them the same kindness and respect that is shown to you. I think we can all agree that the first time we join a class, we are learning and we make mistakes. This happens to teachers as well.

Please use your words wisely. And if you can't, maybe offer a smile of support. We all need time and encouragement to be the best that we can be. Including me.

Beth

# NEW DAY NEW OPPORTUNITY

April 10, 2017

I woke up this morning to the sound of birds and rushing water. The stream behind our home is running at full force and these signs of Spring remind me that every day is a new opportunity to change our lives and circumstances.

Typically exercise classes are quite full at this time of year as we all try to shed those winter pounds and prepare for summer. Each day is full of potential and we can achieve our goals when we remember that what matters is the present moment. Yesterday may have been less than perfect but today we can work to renew our commitments and keep working toward our goals.

While we often meet in classes a few times per week, we may not know the struggles that some fellow gym mates are handling in their personal lives. It is not always easy to get ourselves to class but some clients have added challenges that remind me not to take anything in life for granted. During one of my busiest classes last week, I took a moment to whisper to a client whom I had not seen in a couple of years, how happy I was to see them. It turns out that this client had suffered a stroke. They were so grateful to be back and so full of smiles and joy.

This particular client represents many of us who have had to overcome serious challenges in order to enjoy the simple things in life. Each day is a gift. We must use it wisely because we never know what is in store for us.

Beth

# BE KIND

September 28, 2020

We are all doing our best to survive COVID-19 and I feel that now more than ever, we need to make an effort to be kind. Most of us have not known the type of suffering that is rampant in the world today, and as such we are ill-equipped to deal with the stress that comes with the limitations on our freedom of movement, for example. This is causing us to be unnecessarily rude and short-tempered at times. Last week, I shared a story on Facebook about one of my dear friends and it exemplifies what it means to be kind. I felt I needed to share it more broadly in the hope that this kindness will spread.

My friend found herself in a situation two weeks ago that could have ended very badly but because she chose to be kind and rise above the anger and frustration, everyone was better off in the end.

You see she was waiting in line to pay for her gas after having filled up at the pump, but the customer ahead of her had entered the gas station without a mask and the attendant was refusing to serve this client. An argument was taking place because this particular client only had cash, and because of poor health, was unable to wear a mask. My friend was frustrated with the situation and recognized that the best way to get everyone to settle down would be to simply pay the bill of the unmasked client. The client finally exited the gas station so that things could move forward and then the client tried to pay my friend who understandably didn't want to take the cash for fear of exposure to a stranger.

We could be angry with the mask-less client. "She should know better!" But we don't know what she is dealing with.

We could be angry with the gas attendant. "Come on, show some sympathy." But his/her job is probably on the line if this rule is broken.

We could think my friend crazy. "Why would you give away your money like that?"

Or we could simply recognize the kindness that my friend displayed and ask ourselves how we might step in to help two people move past a difficult situation, so that the world will be a better place for all of us.

Have a great day everyone and let's all remember that none of us are experts at this pandemic experience. We are all doing our best and most of us need a hand right now more than ever.

Beth

# GET YOUR MIND INTO THE GAME

January 16, 2019

When we launched our winter session at the gym last week, I noticed that many of my students were missing out on a very important aspect of exercise. I call it 'auto-pilot' syndrome. People show up in class, willing and ready to participate but I can tell that their minds are elsewhere. People tend to go through the motions physically, without really connecting their mind to what they are doing with their bodies.

It is my job to pull you back into the present moment during our time together and that is why I raise or lower my voice occasionally. Heck, I have even started to growl at times while cueing just to snap my clients out of their daze. FYI, sometimes I am concerned that a student might injure themselves or others because they are distracted.

To get the full benefit we need to tune in to what we are doing every minute of our workout. For instance, when I call 'football' during aerobics, I have asked people to hold their hands around an imaginary ball. I started doing this because my clients were hanging their arms limp by their sides, and in many cases, barely moving their feet. Instead, let's imagine that you are making that million dollar salary and carry that ball as far as you can go!

We will achieve what we believe. You are in charge of your fitness and you can have a positive impact on your health by really tuning your mind into your activities. That is why I try to prompt your thoughts with suggestions throughout the class, especially during Essentrics®. I need you to imagine a resistance because we do not use weights in that class but we use our imaginations to 'push that piano or grab that elastic or lift that feather.'

There is only so much I can do as your trainer. I want you to succeed at achieving your goals and much of that is about your ability to use your mind to get over the finish line. It is true that we don't always feel like exercising and I am the first to congratulate all of my students for getting their butts to class.

The days are shorter and there are many reasons why our thoughts are elsewhere, however I hope to encourage you to focus on the task at hand, no matter where you are or what you are doing. You will achieve results that much quicker and easier if you fully engage your mind in your activities. Please leave your To-Do list at the door and really try to think about the cues you are hearing and how the moves are helping to make you stronger, more flexible and balanced.

Beth

# ATTITUDE IS EVERYTHING

February 1, 2017

So much in our lives is out of our control. Situations arise and we have to deal with them whether we like it or not. I meet people every day who have been told by their doctor that they have to get to the gym to improve their physical condition before things deteriorate further. Once this type of client has joined my class, I make it my mission to make their experience joyful.

Many clients are dealing with chronic knee, hip and shoulder pain. Doctors will often insist that someone start attending the gym before surgery to improve the recovery process. Building up the muscles around the injury site speeds recovery. Remember that even if you are in constant pain, a positive attitude will go a long way in helping you to achieve your goals. We can choose how we 'show up.'

I too have chronic conditions that flare up at certain times. I have no choice but to show up with a positive attitude and I am thankful for this every single day because I now know that these conditions get worse if my attitude is one of 'woe is me.' A negative thought cycle feeds on itself and it is a downward spiral of ill health and misery. I'm not saying it is easy to 'stay up.' It is bloody hard but if you have managed to get yourself to the gym, when you are in chronic pain already, you are a superhero and have done the hard work. Now take it one step further and watch the magic happen.

Try to be fully present when you are in class. Distract your mind away from the pain by focusing on the task at hand. When you focus fully on the cues of the teacher and the muscles that you're working, you will see a gradual shift in your thought process and once more, you will give your mind a break from worry.

I used to tell people to leave their troubles outside of the door. We all have them but try to enter the class with fresh eyes and an open heart and mind. The physical exercise is just one of the elements of the workout. If you absorb yourself fully in the process, you should feel a sense of mental relief. It can feel like you have had a vacation in the sense that your regular routine has changed.

Please know that I can tell when your mind is occupied with thoughts other than the task at hand. My concern is for your safety. Distracted thinking leads to loss of footing in the cardio segment which puts you at risk for falling. If your mind is elsewhere, it is not on proper form during the weight lifting segments which can increase your risk of injury, so you will hear me try to pull you out of your reverie with an occasional bad joke. I'm trying to remind you that in this very moment, we are lucky to be together exercising. It is a gift, not a chore. See it this way and watch your attitude improve your life.

Beth

# PARTIES ARE GOOD FOR YOUR HEALTH

. December 12, 2018

I host a few Christmas parties each season for my students to show my appreciation for the support that they give to me over the year. It is no secret that I love my job and I love being able to share this time of celebration. It is basically just an excuse to get together and share good food and lots of laughter. Today, as I was hosting my fourth student gathering (a nice breakfast after our workout), it hit me how important relationships are at the gym.

I can honestly say that the students who take the time to make friends and form bonds are the ones who benefit the most from their experience at the gym. I can see first hand the positive impact that this social connection has on the clients, especially those who have lost their spouses or those battling disease or chronic pain. This bonding makes my students more inclined to get themselves to the gym even when they feel down, and once they arrive and are among friendly faces, the magic happens. They begin to forget their troubles for a while and in that time, I get the body moving and the blood flowing which enhances the good feelings even more!

Exercise is easier to do when we are among friends and the same is true for most things in life. My goal is to get you to keep coming back to the gym. Facilitating the formation of friendships by hosting a party or two every year gives me a better chance at being successful. We all win!

I hope you are getting an opportunity to share some joy with friends this season. Ask someone out for a coffee after class and get to know each other. The rewards can be everlasting!

Beth

# JUST SAY "NO!"

August 9, 2016

Balance can be hard to achieve if you are the kind of person who says "Yes," to everyone and everything. Learning to express our sentiments clearly is beneficial to our health. My son is living proof.

Josh is a determined and wise young man. When he visits, we have long chats and during these moments I learn quite a bit about him and myself in the process. Recently he was explaining to me how he handles it when people are demanding too much of his time. "Mom, I have made a habit of saying 'no' instantly. If I really don't want to do something I tell the person right away." He went on to explain that the first few times that he did this, it felt as if he was being a bit mean, but with practice it got easier and he's now happier and more carefree.

I have struggled with being a 'people pleaser,' myself. My desire to impress has often resulted in me being unhappy in jobs or relationships. Thankfully, I recognized this characteristic in myself about three years ago and I am actively working on being more like my son. Josh figured this out at 23, while it has taken me 47 years to piece it together!

The key to speaking our minds is saying it with grace and kindness. At times we may offend people but I have discovered that it is better to be true to ourselves than to live with regret.

See you soon,

Beth

# WHAT'S YOUR PROBLEM?

May 2, 2016

We all have those friends who keep us in line. Those friends who are willing to listen and help us find solutions to our problems. I am lucky that I have a few ladies in my life who help me to keep things in perspective. One lady in particular, who has worked hard to survive cancer over the last two or three years, is quick to look me right in the eye and say, "Well if that is the biggest problem you have right now, then life is good!"

I don't think that she means anything deeper than the actual statement but to have it come from someone who has suffered so greatly, really snaps me out of my whining in a hurry. When someone asks my husband how life is going, he has a cute way of answering. "Well, I feel blessed that my life is simple."

A few years ago, I was in the hospital every single day visiting my sick father. I did this for a year while holding down three jobs and raising three teenagers. My life was not my own. That was tough. We must remember the good going on around us and consider that our situation could be much worse. Even when we are in the hospital, there are opportunities to make someone else's day brighter. There are always others around us who are suffering more. When we look to make things better and act on them, it makes us happier and life better!

I have a fabulous job. I work with wonderful people. My health is top notch at the moment. I live in a peaceful environment. My kids are now adults. They are healthy and happy and on their own for now and my husband and I are looking forward to the next phase of life together.

My hope is that when times get tough, that I keep things in perspective. We have food, shelter, our health and love and nothing else matters. Add up your own reasons to be happy and you will find many I am certain.

We have to choose to focus on the positive and steer clear of negative people and situations. Life is too short to be unhappy, so do your best to shine on those around you and soon you will discover that you have no real problems, only reasons to be happy.

Beth

# FAMILY HISTORY CAN HELP YOU HEAL

August 8, 2016

I've read many books this summer and one of the most interesting was written by Mark Wolynn, *It Didn't Start With You*. The premise behind Mark's book is that the roots of our anxiety, phobias and depression etc., may reside "in the lives of our parents, grandparents and even our great-grandparents" and that "traumatic experience can be inherited."

This book forced me to sit down and really examine my family tree and put myself in the shoes of my ancestors. It has been a fascinating journey so far and I have come to understand the importance of knowing our history.

My grandmother arrived in Canada in 1912 at the age of 12 as one of 100,000 Home Children who were sent to Canada to work on farms. My grandmother went on to forge a wonderful life after her time of service on a farm in the Eastern Townships of Quebec but I can certainly see how this experience shaped my own mother. Granny was abandoned at nine years of age and as such likely developed a very tough exterior. Mark suggests that if we know what happened in our family tree, we can begin to see the ripple effects on subsequent generations. We can start to identify patterns and in so doing, bring about change.

Most families have secrets lurking in the family tree that can help to explain why we are raised a certain way. I encourage anyone struggling with mental health issues to read this book. I discovered that many women in my family have struggled with serious challenges which resolved some questions and made me feel less alone.

Beth

# GIVE YOURSELF A BREAK

October 11, 2017

Most of us want results fast and occasionally I run into a client who wants to give up after only one workout or dance class. I am always shocked when someone walks up to me and says, "Should I just give up?" Knowing that my response could either make or break the fragile person standing in front of me is sobering and occasionally I pause to question whether the experience is causing them too much stress.

The bottom line is we all have to decide what is right for us and if you're leaving every single class feeling deflated and miserable, maybe you need to find another type of exercise program that inspires and motivates you to be your best self. At the same time however, you have to give yourself permission to be imperfect and make mistakes.

You cannot expect to master a new skill after only one hour and if you find something that throws you off balance a bit, that just might be exactly what you need to grow. You showed up in fitness classes because your heart was telling you that you needed to make a change and you can't succeed by running away from the challenge.

It is true that we are hardest on ourselves and perhaps some of us don't like feeling lost or imperfect in front of other people. I guess it all depends on our long term goals. You have to put in the time and the work if you want to change your body composition and improve your dance skills. You will not necessarily get everything correct the first class or for the first few weeks but the reward comes when you stick it out and give yourself time to adapt and grow.

I used to tell my clients to attend at least three classes before giving up. Now I recommend giving it a month or two or the whole 12-week session before giving up. Think about how long it takes a child to learn how to walk. They fall constantly but we never say, "You should just give up!"

Give yourself a break and a hug! Wrap your arms around yourself and squeeze. Give yourself time to make positive changes in your life. You deserve it.

Beth

# JE ME SOUVIENS

January 6, 2016

Do you meditate? Most people smile and admit that though they are interested in meditation, they have never tried. Some people claim that they could never sit still for any length of time.

I take a weekly course on meditation in Montreal. I have been participating since the fall and I have to say that it has become the highlight of my week. We discuss our day briefly and then we are led through a guided meditation that is incredibly effective in relieving stress. It is a wonderful way to wind down after a hard day because it changes our focus by putting an end to the 'stories' that play out in our heads, about what we should have said or done during the day. Simply breathing and getting in tune with our physical selves puts our mind at ease.

Yesterday I was killing time waiting for my course to start by browsing some books on meditation at Chapters. I picked up a book by Thich Nhat Hahn, a Vietnamese Buddhist monk. I flipped through the pages and landed on a paragraph that described one of his visits to Montreal. How amazing was that? As he told the story he mentioned that he had noticed the motto printed on all of our license plates; 'Je me souviens.'

He mentioned to the cab driver that this constant reminder to 'remember' is the perfect way to work meditation practice into daily life. Thich Nhat Hahn suggests that every time our eyes focus on this slogan, we should remember to 'breathe and smile.' The whole idea is to walk through our lives being more mindful of every step. Be grateful for everything that is going well. Many of us have very serious challenges in our lives but no matter how deep our troubles appear to be, there is always some glimmer of hope to build upon. For example, being able to breathe with ease and being able to smile. We take these things for granted.

# GIVE YOURSELF THE TIME TO DREAM

December 2, 2020

I often get told, "you work too much," and to be honest this comment always takes me by surprise because one of my biggest secrets is that I absolutely love teaching fitness and none of what I do feels like work. I used to worry that I looked too happy in my last position and I would try to hide it because so many around me looked so miserable doing their jobs. I often thought to myself, "What to heck is wrong with this picture? Why am I so bloody happy?"

I still don't have an answer as to why others look so unhappy at work but I think I have to come to understand that part of the issue is people settle into a job because it pays the bills and never work toward a better future on the side. Sure I have had some clerical positions that felt like a chore but I have always kept learning and honing my passion in my free time.

And the key is to recognize that your journey is different than anyone else's. I think my constant striving for a better future puts some people off because they are so exhausted carrying their current work load that they cannot imagine doing what I do. But you don't have to do what I do, you need only do what feels right for you. Allow yourself a few minutes each day to work toward a dream that you want to achieve. Ask yourself, if money and time were no object or obstacle, what would you do and then start dreaming.

I reminded my women's circle group yesterday of the old saying, "if you love what you do, you will never work a day in your life." If you are hating your life right now, aside from

COVID, take a deep breath and get quiet within yourself and listen to your heart.

What is it telling you? What lights you up? What could make you want to jump out of bed and get to work on your future?

It starts with a dream.

Beth

# PART NINE

# BETH'S JOURNEY

**A**ssembling five years of blog posts into one book has been like holding up a mirror to myself. The experience has shown me the degree to which I have embraced my profession. I didn't just show up to work each day and put in my time. My objective in spending hours on lesson planning, designing new fitness programs and practicing complex choreography, has always been to improve my ability to teach and help my students to feel successful.

The truth is many trainers make classes so challenging that students feel defeated and discouraged. There is a fine line to walk between designing programs that are good for the student and programs that are good for the trainer. As a PRO TRAINER with canfitpro I encouraged the next generations of instructors to work out for themselves on their own time, and to be fully present for their students when leading classes. "It is not about you; it is about the customer."

As an employee of a fitness facility, I learned early on that in order to keep myself employed I needed to make my students and their success the focal point. I grew weary and bored with trying to be the strongest, fittest person in the room shortly after becoming an instructor. There is a real pressure on new teachers to perform and prove their worth by pushing the participants and themselves to the brink.

While always making sure that I was up to date on my certifications, and that I could teach the class at hand, I decided to become an entertainer of sorts, believing that if I made clients feel good about their fitness experience they would return. I am happy to say that you did return, time and time again, in droves.

One of my fondest memories took place early on in my career when my boss at the time had to open a second fitness class to accommodate the number of students who were on a waiting list to get into my class. She called me at home pretending to be disappointed in me. I was scared to death that I had let her down about something. "I can't believe that you have done this to me!" she exclaimed. "People are complaining that there is only one of you!"

Another fond memory took place when I wanted to introduce line dance to the gym where I worked. My boss agreed to let me give a demonstration session saying that if there was enough interest, I could start a class. The word spread quickly and much to my surprise; 100 students showed up to take part. The staff who take care of security were holding people back from entering the room until I said, "let them all in!" Afterwards, my boss walked into the staff room where I was resting and exclaimed with a big smile on her face, "K, you're fired!" I ended up teaching two levels of dance at that facility for many years and eventually added a private class for advanced students at my own studio.

I have had an amazing journey thus far and I have fond memories of special students who have touched my life personally; however it is important to me that every client who enters my fitness studio knows that they are deeply appreciated. I see you. I recognize the light in you. You matter to me.

The following section of blog posts are personal reflections. I hope that they give you a glimpse of what the class looks like from my point of view.

# A NEW SEASON OF FITNESS

September 14, 2020

Today marks the beginning of a new season of exercise for those of us who are used to fitness classes. Some people are returning to in-person sessions, in a socially distant, mask-wearing way, while others are preferring to exercise outdoors until the weather changes. Luckily, a large number of my former clients have joined me online, and we are continuing our daily Zoom fitness meetings, which have been going on since March 16th! My, how time flies.

I had a lovely two-week holiday this month. I was able to travel within Canada and visit my daughter whom I had not seen in eight months. For those of you with kids you understand how special this was for me and how hard it was to leave her and return to my neck of the woods. The above photo is of a sunrise that takes place ten minutes from her front door. I was so lucky to be able to spend last week on the beach. I even got my first and last sunburn of the season after falling asleep in the warm sun. I really needed to get away and feel the sand beneath my feet before we begin our 12 weeks of fitness together. I hope that you enjoyed your summer. We certainly had a special one with hot weather and wonderful opportunities to meet with friends and family in a safe way outdoors.

As I rushed around preparing my fitness classes today, I couldn't help but remark how this would be the first year in twenty, when I would not be a part of the activities at the Pointe Claire Aquatic Center. Normally, I would have packed my bag the night before, after spending all weekend prepping lesson plans. I would have triple checked that I had my shoes and all that I needed to teach my Monday classes, and then I would have had to leave extra early to fight traffic for at least 90 minutes.

Instead, I walked down the stairs to my in-home fitness studio, and actually breathed a sigh of relief. It was time for a change. The sun has set on my time at the pool, but a new chapter of my life is unfolding.

Life is always changing and shifting and it is best to go with the flow. I am so proud of my students for all that they have mastered about technology in the last six months, and I remain in awe of their determination to keep fit at this time. Bravo!

Beth

# DON'T LOOK FOR PERFECTION HERE

June 1, 2016

I am not perfect. I have never claimed to be perfect. In fact, I have waited in the shadows, letting other people go ahead of me, feeling that they were the perfect ones. Then it occurred to me that I should just be me. Flawed but full of good intentions to share. I will never be all things to all people, so there will always be critics. My time is now. None of us should let the fear of what others may think of us, stop us from living our lives.

Instead of watching life pass me by, I have jumped in full throttle this past year. I have listened to my heart. I have found myself in weird situations and succeeded in turning things around to my advantage. I did not run for cover and hide in the face of challenge. I am making mistakes every single day but guess what? That is where the joy is. I laugh more now than ever before. Putting my unique spin on classes, dances, food and entertainment.

What are you good at? Find ways to spend as much time as possible doing what you love. When you do, you will find happiness. In living my life, instead of dreaming my life from the sidelines, I have met others who are doing the same. We attract exactly what we need, when we need it. We wake up each morning with the chance to take our first steps toward the life that we want. Will you give it a try?

Beth

# YOU ARE MY FOCUS

September 1, 2015

All over the world, trainers are preparing programs for the September start up. I want to let you in on a little secret. When I am designing my classes, you are the focus. I think sometimes we enter classes and already we feel like we will never measure up. That somehow we are failures unless we can keep up to the teacher. Maybe we feel like the teacher is just a paid robot at the front of the class, hired to look good and push people beyond their limits. This is not my goal. I do not want you to become me. I want you to become a healthier version of you!

I want you to enjoy your experience in my class so that you keep coming back. If the class is large, my biggest fear is that beginners will slip through the cracks, feel unnoticed and not return. I want you to know that though I absolutely love my returning students, I have an eye out for the new kid on the block. I will be scoping out the class and trying as hard as I can to connect with the newcomers because I have been that nervous newbie in the back. I know what it is to get up the courage to try a new class and feel goofy in the process. I know how hard it is to find time to get to class. I know that you are busy and so when you appear, it is my mission to let you know that I see you and I am here to serve you!

I do not teach 12-16 classes a week to be the strongest, best performer in the group. I teach that many classes so that I can reach that many people. I want to give a hand up to someone who has just been told that they have diabetes and they have to exercise more. I am there to guide that individual who has been told that they have high cholesterol and high blood pressure and that they have to improve their numbers or their lives are at risk.

Let's face it; some people go to the gym to improve their appearance. While I am also there for those people, what truly motivates me every day is helping people improve their health, combat disease and have fun in the process.

Recently, I have been joking with some of my family and friends, saying that I believe my calling in fitness is to take care of the broken and wounded students. While it is a thrill to help elite athletes be even better, it is ten times more rewarding when a student tells me that because of my class, they are able to get off of medication or that they can now do the things that they love, pain free.

You are my focus and I am ready to help.

Beth

# THANK YOUR CRITICS

June 8, 2015

After successfully completing my fitness instructor training program, this was the answer I received from the first gym that I applied to, "I am sorry but you are not strong enough to teach the nighttime classes!" I was 31 and full of energy and enthusiasm. I had put myself through school in the evenings as my kids were all under five years old. I needed to study at night so I could be at home with them in the daytime.

That man's words crushed me. Especially since I had been attending this small club for many years and was also helping to run the place. I believed that I was a very good teacher up until those words were said to me and then the monster of self doubt began to grow inside of me.

We sometimes forget how powerful words can be. I may have given up my pursuit because of the way that he worded his answer. I wonder how differently my life would have turned out, had I listened to him and given up. Thankfully the lady who trained me needed a substitute to fill in for her during the summer, so I did get my start. I was liked so much that she ended up giving me a class in the evenings. After teaching my first 12-week session, the class was so popular that there was a waiting list to get in! Over 15 years later my classes are full and more importantly my students are healthy and happy.

In retrospect, I do not hold anything against the man who denied me my start. He was simply not good at communicating. He could have chosen a far better way to word his opinion. When I am experiencing one of my many moments of joy while teaching, I often flash back to that meeting and smile and thank him as because of him, I pushed myself to be the best teacher that I could be. I also realized shortly after taking that first job, that it is not my mission to be the 'strongest' person in the room. My mission is to help my students to be their best!

Follow your heart and thank your critics because they can sometimes give us that little bit of magic that separates us from the crowd.

Beth

# MY RESPONSIBILITY

April 19, 2016

I am so lucky that my classes are full. This is wonderful news for someone like me who works so hard to create and deliver quality programming each session. Some gyms hire the teachers but also provide the programs. The teacher is simply responsible for delivering what the boss has designed.

What I am responsible for however is making certain that the room is safe for the clients and part of this is having to manage the large numbers of keen participants! In most gyms you have to pass through a turnstile and show your identification to the reception desk. Our gym is very trusting and once you have paid for one of the four types of memberships, we generally trust that students will attend only the classes within the program that they have paid for.

I am responsible for checking people's membership rights as they enter my class. Now that my numbers are growing I have to count the number of people entering to make sure that the room will be safe and effective for everyone. FYI, I have about two minutes to do all of this.

Should an accident happen in any class, the teacher is the one who will be scrutinised first to make certain that all protocols were followed.

For example, did the clients have the proper foot wear and if not, were they warned that they were at risk? Some clients forget their shoes and want to lift weights when they are barefoot. I have to make sure that they know there is risk involved. Some clients insist on chewing gum or having candy in their mouths while working out. This is a huge choking hazard and it is prohibited in our facility. I check shoelaces etc. Yesterday there was a new client doing aerobics too close to people's bags and he was at risk for tripping, so I had to tell him to move ahead.

I am there early to make sure that fire exits are clear. That the equipment is safe. That the floor is free from debris and that I have all of the equipment that I will need for all of the students who are going to show up.

All to say that my mind is on a million things, not to mention delivering the program that I have designed. So though I do my best to deliver this program with a cheerful smile on my face, if I seem a bit distracted it is because I have a concern within the room. Ultimately we are all there to have fun, exercise and get in shape. I love my job and my students. Thank you to all of my students who help me out in whatever way that they can, be it putting away equipment or greeting new students.

See you soon,

Beth

# MY MOTIVATION

June 22, 2016

It amazes me how excited I still get seeing brand new students achieve success. Many of you were in the first line dance class of the summer session yesterday and saw me giggling with joy. Let me explain. I have many dedicated students who have been with me for years and though I get to see you improving aspects of your fitness, I tend to take it for granted because you are all so capable. I am still happy to watch you succeed but there is nothing like watching a hesitant beginner, with low confidence, come into the class and rise above the challenge, to the point where they are smiling and laughing.

I was teaching a combined level 1 and 2 dance class yesterday which is already a challenge because I have to try to keep the class interesting for each of the levels. Within this complex group of dancers, I then had five students who had never danced before, so I had to keep it simple enough and hope that the beginners would feel fabulous and want to come back, yet interesting for the experienced dancers.

All of the beginners mastered the easier dances after several walls. They started out missing steps but before the song was complete, they had found the beat and were dancing right alongside the experts. This never ceases to make me smile from the inside out! I just cannot get enough of seeing their eyes light up. I get the same feeling watching any of my dancers master a complex dance after several weeks of practice. I was reminded yesterday of just how much I love teaching!

Beth

# MY MISSION

October 18, 2016

I am feeling very proud today. I had to take last week off from teaching to get over bursitis and yesterday was my first day back to class. If you have never had bursitis you should know that it is a painful condition that requires rest. I could not move properly at all. I did exactly what my physio told me to do and I was back to my activities in no time.

I am proud because I have designed all of my programming with 'the injured client' in mind so I was easily able to adapt and thrive in my own class. It sounds as though I am tooting my own horn and I guess I am. I work hard to make my classroom a welcoming environment for all ages and abilities and it was nice to take a fresh look at the result of my labour.

I stopped trying to be the strongest person in the room many years ago and switched my focus to helping my clients be the best that they can be. If your back is sore or you have bad knees, there is a way to train the rest of your body pain free. Sometimes these life injuries can stop us from coming to the gym but really you should ask your trainer to adapt the exercises to suit your needs. Or you should be seeking help from a medical professional or physiotherapist.

The key is to find a way to keep moving.

See you soon,

Beth

# WHY AM I GIVING SO MUCH AWAY?

November 3, 2016

Several people have asked me why I write this blog? They have suggested that I may be giving too much of myself away for free. This is a very real concern and I understand where they are coming from but I do it for two reasons.

1. I have so much practical experience teaching fitness that I feel a responsibility to share my knowledge with others. Yes, I am writing a fitness book and one day I will have it ready for sale but until that time, I want to share my opinions with my current students so that they can benefit today. Yes, someone could be stealing my thoughts and words and be marketing them as their own. Unfortunately this is part of working online. All I can do is live my life with integrity and honesty and hope that my audience is doing the same. The writing on this blog is copyrighted material.

2. Though I hope to be teaching fitness forever, my plan is to transition into a writer. Writing this blog several times a week forces me to put my writing hat on and produce. I have maintained this blog and Better Balance with Beth Oldfield, since April 2015. Most people thought that I would give up after a few weeks but I have loved every minute.

My blogging success has given me the confidence to submit two short stories to a contest. I will find out how I did in April, 2017. This was a huge step for me because I have always been too afraid to share my stories with friends and family. The response has been heartwarming which proves to me that I am on the right path. I was terrified about starting this blog but it has worked out well for me and my students.

"Our greatest life lives on the other side of our fears." – Oprah
We cannot settle but we must keep trying new things.
See you in class.
Beth

# BEST COMPLIMENT

January 17, 2018

Occasionally I hear wonderful things from my students. "Because of your class, I'm in better shape and my life has improved in the following ways" I love knowing that people are meeting their fitness goals and seeing improvement in their health. Your success stories motivate me to keep learning and improving as a teacher. Last week, I received a very different compliment and probably the best one to date. "I became an instructor because of attending your classes!"

I have to admit that these words stopped me in my tracks. When I introduced myself to the new young teacher in our center she looked very familiar. I questioned whether we had met before and she admitted that she used to attend my class many years ago when I taught at night. She pointed out the position in the room that she held for years, and when she smiled I remembered her instantly. At the time, I was new to teaching at approximately 30-34 years old. I was a mom in the daytime to three kids under five and a fitness instructor in the evening.

I officially feel old now but in a good way. I am very touched to know that I helped to motivate someone to become an instructor. This is not an easy business but when you truly love what you do, the experience is incredibly rewarding.

Keep those stories coming. I love knowing how I may have played a role in your fitness journey.

Beth

# I'M IN THE REPAIR BUSINESS

March 20, 2019

I would love to be able to say that students show up in my fitness classes because they LOVE working out! The truth is most people turn to exercise when their doctor tells them that they need to either lose weight or strength train. My goal is to make the experience of fitness enjoyable so that my participants will commit to attending. This will improve their chance for success!

I actually feel as though I am in the repair business, trying to help people 'fix' their bodies. People come up to me regularly and grab their belly or the skin under their arms or their inner thighs or buttocks and say, "Can you fix this?"

I'm happy to help and I love seeing people transform themselves through dedication, hard work and determination! Yes, it is possible to have a positive effect on your health and I love that doctors are prescribing fitness as medicine because in my opinion it is the best option.

Even when we feel that we are in shape, injuries can suddenly appear, seemingly out of the blue. I hear the following almost weekly, "I don't get it. I have been doing this same activity for years with no problem but now I can't!"

Just because we are in good shape does not mean that we will never get injured. I also have to help people understand that change is part of living a healthy life. We cannot expect our bodies to stay in top shape, if we don't train all of the components of fitness equally. We need to train our cardiorespiratory system, our muscular strength and flexibility in a well balanced fashion and our mental health as well because when one of these systems weakens, we put ourself at risk for injury.

We can't always do the same classes and expect the same positive results that we experienced initially. We have to switch up what we are doing regularly to keep our bodies balanced. Moving our bodies in activities that favour just front and backwards movements can result in weaknesses in all of the muscles that are not being used to their true potential. So I get people complaining that they cannot do "xyz" like they used to and I have to remind them that variety is the key to great health. Change is necessary even if it is unwanted.

I myself am dealing with an injury that needs some repair. This minor issue came up five years ago and I have done my best to deal with it successfully but now I realize that I need to change my approach. We are getting older even though we feel great 99% of the time. The key is to listen when our body speaks to us through various aches and pains and make adjustments right away.

I love being in the repair business. We can fix most problems with fitness. Your dedication will pull you through!

See you next week.

Beth

# SMALL PART OF YOUR JOURNEY

November 7, 2018

One of my favourite things as a teacher is having a student come back to my classes after a very long hiatus. I've been teaching for 20 years, so they often have to remind me of when and where we met and what type of exercise we were doing at the time. I enjoy this as I get to take a trip down memory lane and laugh about all of the various forms of fitness that I've done with people. I get to hear what has transpired in their lives in their time away. But one of the hardest things is to watch people go! I get very attached to my clients and because most of my weekly hours are devoted to a gym where I am just an employee, I often have no idea why people stop attending my group fitness classes. This can be hard on me as I am left wondering about their health and why they moved on.

Yesterday, while lamenting about this over lunch, a friend of mine who is a retired social worker, offered me a different perspective. I need to remember that I'm a small part of someone's journey through this life. This doesn't minimize the impact that I have on people, but instead of being sad when students stop attending class, I should be happy for the opportunity that I had to help them along their way. It really is a blessing to be of service to people who are trying to improve their health through fitness. Students are not meant to be with me forever. I need to look at my classroom (gym studio) as a place that people pass through instead of a place where they stay. My wish is to give people the tools they need to live their best lives and for the most part I am succeeding. Thanks Susan!

Beth

# Acknowledgements

First and foremost I must thank my students for believing in me and trusting me with their health. More often than not, my students sign up and pay for their classes without even enquiring about the activity that I have planned. I know that you feel safe and supported and this warms my heart.

I have to thank Peter, my husband, for always supporting my crazy endeavours like transforming our basement into a fully equipped fitness studio in 2007. In 2020 he didn't even blink when I told him I would be using that studio to deliver not just two classes per week (as was the norm) but twelve virtually. This meant that the peace and quiet he normally enjoyed on my days away from home were no more. He has not complained once.

I must thank my editor, Margaret Goldik, who challenges me to follow my dreams. Thanks for keeping my punctuation on point. If there is an extra comma or exclamation point in this book, it is surely my fault!!

And finally, I must thank Suzanne Doyle-Ingram who has published several of my books. Because of you I can tick several boxes off of my bucket list.

My greatest thanks to you all.

Sincerely,

Beth

www.ingramcontent.com/pod-product-compliance
Lightning Source LLC
Chambersburg PA
CBHW072110270326
41931CB00010B/1510